GIVING ADOLESCENTS A VOICE:
CONDUCTING A RAPID ASSESSMENT OF ADOLESCENT HEALTH NEEDS

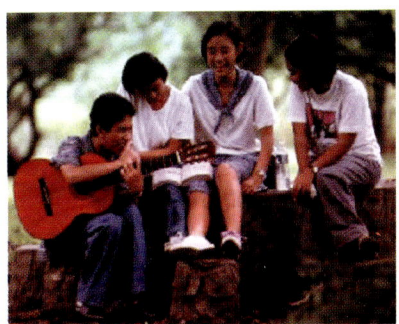

A MANUAL FOR HEALTH PLANNERS AND RESEARCHERS

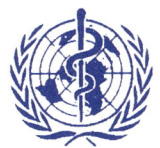

WORLD HEALTH ORGANIZATON
Regional Office for the Western Pacific
Manila, 2001

WHO Library Cataloguing in Publication Data

Giving adolescents a voice : conducting a rapid assessment of adolescent health needs : a manual for health planners and researchers

1. Adolescence.
2. Health services needs and demands – methods.
3. Needs assessment – methods.
4. Manuals.
I. World Health Organization. Regional Office for the Western Pacific.

ISBN 92 9061 159 6

The World Health Organization welcomes requests for permission to reproduce or translate its publications, in part or in full. Applications and enquiries should be addressed to the Office of Publications, World Health Organization, Geneva, Switzerland or to the Regional Office for the Western Pacific, Manila, Philippines, which will be glad to provide the latest information on any changes made to the text, plans for new editions, and reprints and translations already available.

© World Health Organization 2001

Publications of the World Health Organization enjoy copyright protection in accordance with the provisions of Protocol 2 of the Universal Copyright Convention. All rights reserved.

The designations employed and the presentation of the material in this publication do not imply the expression of any opinion whatsoever on the part of the Secretariat of the World Health Organization concerning the legal status of any country, territory, city or area or of its authorities, or concerning the delimitation of its frontiers or boundaries.

The mention of specific companies or of certain manufacturers' products does not imply that they are endorsed or recommended by the World Health Organization in preference to others of a similar nature that are not mentioned. Errors and omissions excepted, the names of proprietary products are distinguished by initial capital letters.

TABLE OF CONTENTS

List of Boxes	v
Foreword	vii
Introduction to the Manual	1
Rapid Assessments for Health Planning	1
Rapid Assessment Procedures	1
Content of the Manual: A Range of Ingredients, Not a Recipe Book	2
Who is this Manual For?	3
Benefits and Limitations of Rapid Assessments	3
Organization of the Manual	4
Adolescent Health Needs and National Development	4
Part I Conducting an Adolescent Health Needs Rapid Assessment: Steps in Implementation	9
Introduction to Part I	11
Steps in Conducting a Rapid Assessment	12
Step 1 – Establishing the Core Research Team	13
Step 2 – Setting Objectives and Conducting a Literature Review	15
Step 3 – Constructing a Theme List	17

Step 4 – Choosing Methods	21
Step 5 – Constructing Topics for Free Listing, Check-lists and Question Guides	25
Step 6 – Deciding on Sampling, Location and Responsibility	33
Step 7 – Entering the Field	38
Step 8 – Data Management and Analysis	40
Step 9 – Preparation of the Report	43
Summary: Guiding Principles for Undertaking Rapid Assessments	46
Part II An Overview of Rapid Assessment Methods: What they are and how to use them	51
Introduction to Part II	52
Some Tips on Conducting Interviews and Discussions	53
Review of Secondary Data	55
Community Meetings	57
Key Informant Interviews	60
Focus Group Discussions	63
In-depth Interviews	67
Observation	70
Mapping by Researchers	72
Social Mapping	73
Free Listing	75
Pile Sorting	78
Pile Sorting (1): Conducting a Rating Exercise	78
Pile Sorting (2): Conducting a Grouping Exercise	79
Appendix I. Suggested References on Qualitative Research and Rapid Assessment Methods	80
Appendix II. Workshop Programme to develop a Rapid Assessment Protocol	83

LIST OF BOXES

Box 1.	Model of Project Aims and Objectives	15
Box 2.	Discussion Tool for Generating a Theme List for an Adolescent Health Needs Assessment	18
Box 3.	Model of Theme List (with Related Issues)	19
Box 4.	Typical Methods for Rapid Assessments	21
Box 5.	Example of a Main Theme, Related Issues and Possible Data Collection Methods	22
Box 6.	Table of Theme List and Potential Methods of Data Collection	23
Box 7.	Topics for Free Listing (in question format)	26
Box 8.	Example of an FGD Check-list and Question Guide for Adolescents	28
Box 9.	Example of a Check-list and Question Guide for In-depth Interviews with Adolescents	30
Box 10.	Example of a Check-list and Question Guide for Interviews with Key Informants	32
Box 11.	General Suggestions on Sampling	34
Box 12.	A Model of Planned Field Operations	36
Box 13.	A Fieldwork Plan	37
Box 14.	Generic Guide for Preparation of Adolescent Health Needs Assessment Report	43
Box 15.	Tips for Interviews and Discussions	54
Box 16.	Secondary Data Review Guide and Check-list	56
Box 17.	Community Meeting Invitation List Used at Team Headquarters in Viet Nam	58
Box 18.	Check-list for Community Meetings	59
Box 19.	Managing 'Difficult' FGD Participants	66

ACKNOWLEDGEMENT

Principal contributors to the manual were Dr Martha Morrow, Senior Lecturer; Dr Pascale Allotey, Senior Lecturer; Professor Lenore Manderson, Director; and Professor Emeritus Pertti Pelto, Principal Fellow, Key Centre for Women's Health in Society, WHO Collaborating Centre, Department of Public Health, The University of Melbourne, Australia.

Design and desktop publishing were by John Litaridis and Elisa Miotti, Key Centre for Women's Health in Society.

The principal contributors are indebted to colleagues in the collaborative Adolescent Health Needs Assessment Project from the Health Information and Education Center of Ho Chi Minh City, Vietnam, and the Public Health Department of Beijing Medical University, China, for useful suggestions and feedback.

FOREWORD

No longer children, not yet adults – adolescents are at a stage of rapid development when they acquire new capacities and are faced with many new situations. As adolescents face the challenges of the second decade of life, a little help can go a long way in channelling their energy towards positive and productive paths. Neglect of adolescents can lead to problems, both immediately and in the years ahead. One of the most important commitments a country can make for future economic, social and political progress and stability is to address the health and development needs of its adolescents (WHO 1999:212-13).

The World Health Organization Regional Office for the Western Pacific recognizes the critical importance of enhancing adolescent (10-19 years old) well-being. However, a serious weakness in current health planning is the lack of knowledge about, and contact with, the adults of tomorrow. Research models often fail to involve and engage adolescents themselves, thus failing to gauge their perspectives properly. As a population, adolescents are notoriously difficult to study. Shyness, lack of self-awareness, undeveloped communication skills and the generation gap create special difficulties for researchers and programme planners, most of whom have left their own youth far behind. These difficulties are more pronounced when there are further gaps related to class, gender, or geographic origin.

Health planning should involve not just problem solving but the full development of individuals and societies. This manual was developed during 1999 and 2000 under the sponsorship of the WHO Regional Office for the Western Pacific. Its purpose is to support governments in understanding more fully the health problems confronting today's adolescents, and the opportunities that exist for working in partnership with young people to help them reach their full potential. An early version was designed in 1999 by a multidisciplinary team at the Key Centre for Women's Health in Society, a WHO Collaborating Centre at The University of Melbourne, Australia. Staff at the Key Centre worked with researchers in Viet Nam (Health Information and Education Center, Ho Chi Minh City) and China (Public Health Department, Beijing Medical University) to develop protocols for rapid assessments, and to field-test the manual. Both national teams conducted regional assessments. The manual was modified in mid-2000 on the basis of field experiences in both countries.

The aim of the manual is to aid the implementation of a national-level rapid assessment of adolescent health needs. The focus is on giving young people a voice through participatory techniques, thereby providing useful evidence for the development of appropriate adolescent health policies and programmes. We commend this manual to health ministries in our region, and look forward to future collaboration in the interests of adolescents. We believe a commitment to our young people will enhance prospects for development, peace and well-being throughout our region.

Shigeru Omi, M.D., Ph.D.
Regional Director
World Health Organization
Western Pacific Region

INTRODUCTION TO THE MANUAL

Rapid assessments for health planning

Shrinking national health budgets, organizational change in response to health reforms, and the sheer size and complexity of current threats to health present major challenges to health officials. In order to target interventions equitably and appropriately, governments must be able to identify and prioritize health problems based on available evidence. In addition, health programmes are more successful when the target population is involved in the identification of needs.

Many health ministries lack sufficient funds to conduct large-scale epidemiological surveys. In any case, these often fail to illuminate social, cultural, environmental and economic influences on health and health behaviours. Lengthy qualitative investigations can explore these areas, but are time-consuming and costly, and their findings cannot necessarily be generalized to the wider population. **Rapid health needs assessments** offer a useful alternative, and are employed increasingly as a cost-effective, participatory tool for health planning.

Rapid assessment procedures

Rapid assessment procedures (RAP) have been used increasingly for data gathering and evaluation in health. They share some common features with *rapid rural appraisal* (RRA), first developed for agricultural development, and *participatory rural appraisal* (PRA), the main aim of which is 'to generate information for action rather than for the advancement of knowledge as in basic research' (Campbell et al. 1999: 53). RAPs draw upon a variety of research tools (both qualitative and quantitative) to investigate problems.

A rapid health needs assessment is not itself a *method* of data gathering, but an *approach* to data gathering that makes strategic use of existing methods, encouraging faster data collection, data analysis and reporting for the purposes of health planning. It is inherently participatory, and can be conducted by a team with different levels of research experience. It cannot fully replace time-intensive investigations, but can offer important contextual information and shed light on motivations, beliefs and knowledge of a diverse range of individuals and groups.

Health needs assessments reveal the **gap** between existing services and those desired or needed by a target population. The assessment of what is *desired* comes from the voices of the target group. The assessment of what is *needed* draws on external perspectives (e.g. from key informants or observational studies) and review of secondary data.

Content of the manual: a range of ingredients, not a recipe book

As the name suggests, rapid assessments are intended to be undertaken rapidly, and so we emphasize practicality. This manual provides a staged approach to develop and conduct a national-level adolescent health needs rapid assessment. In this manual we:

- ❖ Provide a brief overview of adolescent health
- ❖ Offer a variety of methods and tools as options for data gathering
- ❖ Provide illustrations of planning tools
- ❖ Describe specific strategies to assist field implementation
- ❖ Provide cases from field experience

This manual is designed as a flexible guide, not a rigid blueprint. It offers the research team a wide range of tools. It does not prescribe which ones should be adopted, because issues, cultures, populations, research expertise, budgets and available time vary from country to country. Choosing methods, and deciding sampling can be done only by the team within the local context.

Who is this manual for?

This manual is for use by those undertaking a national-level rapid assessment of adolescent[1] health needs. A national level needs assessment, by its very nature, can sample only very selected parts of the rich diversity in any nation. By selecting particular target regions, localities, and special populations, the data gathering methods can capture major variations related to local environment or individual life situation.

This manual can be used to conduct regional or local-level needs assessments, with some adaptation, but we assume that the approach will be national or cross-regional.

We also assume that assessment results will lead to programme or policy development. Hence, the approach stresses collecting data for action, not simply for theorizing. The methods described can also be used for monitoring and evaluating adolescent health programmes, but in this manual, the focus is on identification of needs.

Benefits and limitations of rapid assessments

Rapid assessments are used to gain a quick insight into the needs of a particular community, and produce findings that can be translated into action. The approach consists of a variety of methods, mainly qualitative, for gaining rich, in-depth perspectives on complex issues.

Because qualitative approaches use non-random, mainly purposive, sampling strategies, and because of the unstructured nature of the tools themselves, results cannot be generalized to the entire target population. This limitation can be minimized partially by *triangulation* of data sources, that is, the use of several methods, and collation of existing epidemiological and other secondary data. 'Triangulation is a powerful way to assess the validity of results' (Campbell et al. 1999: 29), and we recommend it strongly here. Nonetheless, reports and recommendations based upon rapid assessments should explicitly note the study limitations.

---

[1] WHO defines adolescents as those in the 10-19 age group.

Organization of the manual

Part I summarizes the basic steps for conducting an adolescent health needs rapid assessment, from the establishment of a Core Research Team to production of a report. Within this section, we provide examples for undertaking the assessment, and guiding principles for adaptation to local circumstances. Points of decision, and how they can be considered, are also described.

In **Part II**, we provide an overview of methods of data gathering and management as guides to field implementation. This overview is only a summary of key points, and not a complete training guide. Useful tips and cautions are included to assist any new team members, or as reminders for more experienced members. We assume that researchers will have familiarity with most, if not all, methods before beginning the assessment. Some recommended references on qualitative methods and on rapid assessment techniques are listed in **Appendix I**.

Appendix II describes a 10-day schedule that can be used by teams to develop a plan to conduct the rapid assessment in an individual country. This schedule was used in Viet Nam and China for this purpose.

Adolescent Health Needs and National Development

Today, more than half of the world's populatiopn is below the age of 25 and four out of five young people live in developing nations. To a large extent, the future prosperity of countries will depend on having a healthy and economically productive population. Yet among health professionals, adolescent health has only recently emerged as an international issue.

The upsurge in attention may be influenced by two factors: the size of the cohort and the rise in morbidity and mortality linked to emerging communicable and non-communicable conditions, such as HIV/STIs, injuries, substance abuse, depression and self-harm.

In this sense, both the demographic and health transitions lead to a new focus on adolescent health. Countries stand to reap a "demographic bonus" if this cohort carries good health and professional skills into adulthood, or to acquire greater public deficits if they do not (UNFPA 1998; WHO 1999).

> *A better understanding of adolescent health needs and their potential, along with the principles of effective intervention, disseminated at all levels of society in each culture, and drawn from each culture, can have a powerful influence in developing positive action and fulfilling the enormous potential that the health and development of young people represents both for themselves and for the future of their societies (WHO 1999:22)*

The notion of 'adolescence' as a defined and discrete life phase is a relatively new concept. It is related to earlier sexual maturity, delayed marriage, changing constructions of gender, and a need for greater preparation for the social and economic complexities of adulthood in the contemporary world (UNFPA 1998).

Many adolescents are coming of age in an often dangerous environment. Rapid social change and development are associated with new health risks, as traditional norms, relationships and societal patterns are challenged and transformed. Commercial pressures can exacerbate these risks by presenting life-threatening behaviours and lifestyles as appealing.

These dangers are magnified by the special characteristics of adolescence. Rapid physical growth often outstrips emotional maturity, and peer pressure may override common sense. Gender role expectations, feelings of curiosity and invulnerability — or, conversely, hopelessness linked to economic or social insecurity — may lead to risk-taking (Michell and Amos 1997).

A global teenage culture has emerged in the past half-century, particularly in urban centres, but it is too early to predict whether these external shifts are transient fashions or symbols of more lasting changes in social values (Caldwell *et al.* 1998). Therefore, it is important that countries explore and monitor the needs of their own adolescent populations, and not rely on assumptions about commonalities or differences.

Research exploring adolescent perspectives is rare outside the area of HIV-prevention in most countries (WHO 1999), and even within this field, research designs are often superficial and unconnected with wider issues of sexuality, contraception and gender relations (Efroymson *et al.* 1997). The complex and delicate process of self-understanding and development is poorly integrated in many health promotion programmes for adolescents, for whom sexuality is only one of many, perhaps more compelling, concerns.

An overemphasis on reproductive or sexual health for adolescents ignores widespread behaviours and risks that, in many countries, are more likely to result in premature death and illness. These include smoking, drinking, depression, and dangerous use of motorized vehicles (WHO 1998a, b). It should also be remembered that many adolescents do not engage in any risk behaviours, but we know little about this large cohort.

Effective public health approaches must be based on reliable data that reveal the levels of risk, as well as the perceptions, beliefs and concerns of the target population (Dowsett and Aggleton 1997). Health planning also requires current information about existing health services, including the scope of available human and material resources, and the perspectives and attitudes of health providers themselves. Indeed, it is worth questioning the appropriateness of an illness model for adolescent health policy formulation.

If we adopt a broader definition of health, we will recognize that adolescent health should involve providing curative services, and also opportunities and support to assist young people to develop fully within their societies.

Positive attributes such as self-esteem and resilience, which are associated with health promotion or good health, must be built through multisectoral policies and programmes that nurture adolescents as a group and as individuals. Successful health promotion for adolescents will be evident not only in morbidity and mortality profiles, but in the health habits, life skills and creative energy of young people.

Health planning for adolescents should begin with collecting information about the way adolescents see their own health needs. In addition, other sources are important to gain further insight into needs or risks that may not be visible to adolescents themselves. It is important that researchers know how to listen to adolescents (and other relevant stakeholders) and know what questions to ask. An understanding of adolescent health needs will assist in the development of curative

Focusing only on prevention singles out high-risk groups, thereby dividing young people and reinforcing stereotypes. The promotion of development involves commitment to young people in general ... (WHO 1999: 17).

services, risk-reduction strategies, and preventive health activities, and will also underpin the evolution of programmes and policies that assist young people to become resilient, creative, resourceful, productive and connected to their community and society. The well-being of this population, as well as the well-being of communities and countries, will require nothing less.

This manual is a guide to planning and conducting an adolescent health rapid needs assessment, to produce data for more effective health programmes and policies for the youth of today, and the adults of tomorrow.

PART I

CONDUCTING AN ADOLESCENT HEALTH NEEDS RAPID ASSESSMENT: STEPS IN IMPLEMENTATION

INTRODUCTION TO PART I

In Part I, we describe the steps involved in developing and conducting an adolescent health needs rapid assessment. We first highlight the assumptions and central features of rapid assessments, then offer suggestions about the establishment and composition of research teams. We define the usual parameters in developing such protocols, and identify the aspects that need to be considered when arriving at points of decision. We also summarize the key issues related to data collection, data management and analysis, and offer guidance on preparing a report based on assessment findings.

Within this part, we have included working models as illustrations of various steps and decision points in preparation for the rapid assessment. These models are intended to bring to life the theoretical discussions in the manual, and serve as a stimulus to local decision-making. What is useful or appropriate in one country may be of no benefit in another. Only the spirit or approach of a rapid assessment should be seen as universal; local considerations will influence which methods are used, where, with whom, and in what time-frame.

Throughout Part I we have highlighted key points at which decisions must be made by national teams. These points are marked as follows:

» **DECISION POINT**

These decisions transform the generic protocol into a genuine protocol intended for use within a specific country and setting. In discussing implementation steps, as well as specific methods (see Part II), we have also provided some boxes containing **TIPS** (suggestions you may find helpful) and **CAUTIONS** (possible pitfalls and how to avoid them). These are based upon field experiences in testing the protocol in Viet Nam and China.

Steps in Conducting a Rapid Assessment

In Part I we identify and describe the key components and stages of the rapid assessment. These are listed below, with page numbers for easy reference.

- **Step 1** Establishing the Core Research Team *(p. 13)*
- **Step 2** Setting Objectives and Conducting a Literature Review *(p. 15)*
- **Step 3** Constructing a Theme List *(p. 17)*
- **Step 4** Choosing Methods *(p. 21)*
- **Step 5** Constructing Topics for Free Listing, Check-lists and Question Guides *(p. 25)*
- **Step 6** Deciding on Sampling, Location and Responsibility *(p. 33)*
- **Step 7** Entering the Field *(p. 38)*
- **Step 8** Data Management and Analysis *(p. 40)*
- **Step 9** Preparation of the Report *(p. 43)*

STEP 1

Establishing the Core Research Team

Once a decision has been made to conduct a rapid assessment, a Core Research Team should be established at the national level. Other, secondary members will be recruited as needed in the field, but the Core Research Team will be responsible for planning and implementation. The process by which members are identified will be determined by the organization requesting the needs assessment, but some suggested guidelines follow.

Ideally, the Team should include individuals with several years of research experience, both qualitative and quantitative, with in-depth knowledge of adolescents and/or adolescent health, and with good networks of contacts in other parts of the nation. However, skills in qualitative research are not equally developed in all countries, and adolescent health is a new issue. Therefore, try to include people with experience in at least one area, perhaps inviting short-term input in other areas from other individuals. There should be enough people to carry out all the tasks, too. Membership should be based not only on affiliation and skills, but also on ability to commit to the project. It is important to consider:

- appropriate institutional affiliation (able to represent broad and important interests);
- representation from major ethnic groups and geographic regions;
- multidisciplinary background, including some with expertise in qualitative methods;
- gender balance.

Size of the Team

The size of the Core Research Team depends partly on the intended scope and duration of the assessment. If many regions are being surveyed simultaneously, the Team should be larger than if fewer regions are being surveyed, or if field visits are being conducted consecutively. In the case of a large, simultaneous assessment, it may be necessary to have approximately 6-10 members, while in consecutive assessment, 4-7 members may suffice. The Team leader should have final responsibility for decision-making and submission of the report, but all members should share in all steps of the assessment.

Planning and Preparation Meeting of the Team

As soon as the Team can be assembled, it should meet for approximately 7-10 days to plan the assessment and prepare for fieldwork (Steps 2-7). During this period, Team members should read the manual and take time to practise any new or unfamiliar methods.

Note: In Appendix II is a suggested format and timeframe for a workshop to develop the protocol and prepare for the assessment (Steps 2-7).

TIP

Skilled, knowledgeable people are often busy people. Be sure Core Research Team members have been given sufficient time release from normal duties to devote to the assessment, and that they and their supervisors understand likely time-frames and travel requirements.

STEP 2 — Setting Objectives and Conducting a Literature Review

>> **DECISION POINT**
Decide on objectives for the rapid assessment

Setting Objectives

Every research project needs a set of clear aims and objectives. The Core Research Team should identify these as a first priority, as they will guide all subsequent decisions. Aims and objectives may be influenced by external considerations, including budget and time-frame. It is impossible to find out everything you may wish to know about a given topic or population, so you need to decide upon priorities. In the box opposite, we show a set of generic aims and objectives.

Box 1. Model of Project Aims and Objectives

Project Aim:

This rapid assessment aims to contribute to the development of adolescent health policies and programmes by describing adolescents' own perceived health needs, and their health needs as determined by reviewing information from a variety of external sources.

Specific project objectives are to:

- identify gaps between expressed health desires, objectively determined needs, and existing services for adolescents;

- consider options for structures, programmes and activities to reduce risk, enhance health, and foster environments in which adolescents can achieve their full potential.

Conducting a Literature Review

All research projects should be grounded in available evidence relating to the topic of investigation. Hence, a review should be undertaken by the Team to determine what is already known about adolescent health in your country, and what issues may be of relevance to you.

Try to obtain national data on demographic profiles of adolescents (e.g. size of cohort, literacy levels by region, health patterns and status), and relevant publications or reports from health departments, universities and non-governmental organizations in your country. It is also helpful to look at publications from other countries, including international journals, if these are available.

Conducting a good literature review takes time. Given that this is a rapid assessment, this step may be shortened, but it should not be eliminated entirely. Secondary data reviews are also used to help contextualize findings, and to improve the validity of interpretations and conclusions, and are incorporated into the final report. For this project, secondary data should be reviewed before, during and after primary data collection.

STEP 3
Constructing a Theme List

To conduct qualitative research, it will help if you develop a preliminary Theme List to guide the data collection, as well as data analysis. *Themes* are sometimes called *Topics* or *Categories*, and are the issues, areas, or concepts that are important in understanding adolescent health needs.

Themes can also be seen as the potential *explanations* for or *influences* on health problems. For example, a study about maternal nutrition might identify themes such as cultural beliefs about food, food distribution in the family, time available for shopping/cooking, and cost of food relative to income.

A theme list for this project would include the topics of *direct* research interest (e.g. adolescent health concerns; content of existing services, etc.) along with the ***indirect*** or ***underlying*** influences on health problems or health needs (e.g. social influences on risk behaviour, such as gender norms, poor health status due to chronic malnutrition, effect of isolation on access to treatment options, etc.).

In qualitative research, the Theme List continues to evolve as data are collected and initial findings are discussed in the field. The Team should start, therefore, with a ***preliminary*** Theme List, to which you will add ***emerging*** themes as they arise from data collection and analysis. Bearing in mind the need to keep an open mind in qualitative research, the Theme List should never be seen as final, but rather as a dynamic framework to assist in project focus. Rapid assessment methods are particularly good at exploring concepts and issues that are new to the research team.

The Project Objectives and Theme List build a platform for making central decisions about target groups, samples and methods. Developing these also serves to strengthen shared understandings within the Team, and assists in bringing a clear focus to group discussions.

Make sure you set aside sufficient time to brainstorm themes, during which a large number may be generated, and to arrange and refine them into a list of manageable size. Remember to invite and welcome contributions from all Team members, to take full advantage of their expertise and insights.

To assist in this brainstorming process, we offer a Discussion Tool **(Box 2)** used during adaptation in Viet Nam and China. When using this tool, all members should be encouraged to reflect upon their memories of adolescence as well as their professional knowledge base, both theoretical and practical. A facilitator should be chosen to encourage discussion and keep it on track. We suggest you use large sheets of paper or whiteboard to assist in the process. It is also important to remind the Team of the project objectives.

Box 2. Discussion Tool for Generating a Theme List for an Adolescent Health Needs Assessment

Discussion Topics

- *How do people understand adolescence? Should it be a distinct life phase? Consider this topic in relation to the following:*
    - Memories of your own adolescence
    - As a parent
    - As a researcher
    - As a health educator
    - As a health service provider
    - As a teacher
    - In community work
    - Other

- *What are the special characteristics of adolescence?*
    - How do these affect health needs and service provision?
    - Why is it difficult for adults to understand adolescent needs?

- *How do you think health policy-makers or health programme designers view adolescence?*

- *How have adolescent health issues changed in recent years?*
    - How has service provision changed and why?

- *What youth health issues arise among different populations?*
    - Ethnic minority groups
    - In-school/out-of-school
    - Groups at special risk
    - Urban/rural/isolated
    - Male/female

- *Do you think it will be useful to do a needs assessment in this field (are there any limitations)?*

- *Listing exercise:*
    - List the key health issues, problems and service needs for adolescents today

- *Final exercise:*
    - Try to reduce the list by clustering similar or related themes.

Many themes will be identified during this activity. The final step is to refine or arrange these themes. Decide which themes can be clustered together, and then decide which of these are 'main' themes, and which are 'related issues'. An example of this process, developed in Viet Nam, is presented in **Box 3**.

> **» DECISION POINT** *Develop and organize a theme list*

Box 3. Model of Theme List (with Related Issues)

Theme	Related Issues
Demographic profile of adolescents	Proportion of the total population; urban/rural differences Proportion in-school at different ages in different regions Literacy, joblessness and marriage by age and sex
Health status of adolescents	Morbidity and mortality for this cohort Identification of major causes of morbidity and mortality Reproductive health status of adolescents *(pregnancy, abortion, STIs)*
Adolescent health concerns	Adolescents' perceived health concerns and concepts of health Adolescent health concerns as perceived by others (health planners, youth leaders, teachers, health professionals)
Content and nature of existing adolescent health policies and programmes	National health policies relevant to adolescents Rules and regulations affecting adolescent access and services *(e.g. on sexuality education, contraception, abortion)* Adolescents as target cohort in national, provincial, district or village level policies/programmes

Box 3. Model of Theme List (with Related Issues) (continued...)

Theme	Related Issues
Adolescent health information needs	Perceived information needs of adolescents Adolescent information needs identified by others *(health planners, youth leaders, teachers, health professionals)*
Content, nature and use of existing health services for adolescents	Types of services at various levels Content of services in terms of aims, human and fiscal resources, location Services used by adolescents, and usage patterns Perceptions of services and service needs by adolescents Service needs as perceived by others
Health risks of adolescents	Population patterns of known risk behaviours, including 'high-risk' groups Beliefs and perceptions about risks among adolescents themselves and among others
Cultural, ethnic and geographical influences	Cultural beliefs, customs, language use influencing health risk and health-seeking behaviours (ethnic differences) Role of family in health promotion *(positive or negative)* Impact of geographical factors *(e.g. isolation, terrain, water quality and use, natural disasters)* on risk and services
Impact of economic status and employment	Absolute and relative poverty for various population cohorts Employment levels and wages for out-of-school youth Disposable income/spending patterns for youth in different environments Occupational health issues for adolescents

Source: Adapted from United Nations Population 1997. Population and Reproductive Health Programmes: Applying Rapid Anthropological Assessment Procedures. Technical Report No. 39. UNFPA, New York.

STEP 4 Choosing Methods

In rapid assessments, as in all research projects, the method you select will affect the quality of the project; hence, this stage should be undertaken with great care, and with appropriate expertise. Rapid assessments commonly draw upon a wide range of methods, partly to enable data collection from diverse sources and populations, and partly to strengthen the validity of findings (through triangulation).

Box 4. Typical Methods for Rapid Assessments

> Review of secondary data
>
> Free listing (with sorting and rating)
>
> Social mapping
>
> Mapping by researchers
>
> Observation
>
> Focus group discussions (FGDs)
>
> In-depth interviews
>
> Key informant interviews
>
> Community meetings

Because a particular theme can often be investigated by more than one method, it is important at the outset to brainstorm a full list of potential methods for each. The level of expertise in the Team, or time/budgetary limitations, will determine the final choice.

Below is a list of methods commonly used in rapid assessments.

We recommend that the Core Research Team should select the methods as a group (or in subgroups), using the **Theme List** as a stimulus and guide. *For a description of methods, and summary of their advantages and limitations for an adolescent health needs assessment, see Part II.*

Finally, you should develop a table listing main themes, related issues, and, beside each, all appropriate methods of collecting data.

As an example, we illustrate in **Box 5** just one possible theme (adolescent health concerns), related issues, and a list of potential methods of gathering data on this theme. This process should be followed for each main theme.

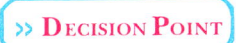

>> DECISION POINT *Construct a table of potential methods to explore each theme*

Box 5. Example of a Main Theme, Related Issues and Possible Data Collection Methods

Main Theme	Related Issues	Data Collection Methods
Adolescent health concerns	Adolescents' perceptions and concerns about health	Free listing ratings Health providers or youth activities FGDs In-depth interviews Secondary data
	Adolescent health concerns as perceived by others (health planners, youth leaders, teachers, health professionals)	Community meetings Key informant interviews

TIP

Remember, decisions about methods here are not final. They may be modified during planning of the fieldwork timetable, or during fieldwork itself, because unexpected difficulties—and opportunities—may arise. The key is to know about a range of methods, understand the limitations and advantages of each, and be flexible when the situation requires a change.

The table you develop will be the main reference document for the project. It will help Team members to monitor their progress in the field, note the richness of data on each theme, identify continuing gaps, and consider new strategies to address them.

Below we offer, as an illustration, a full table including theme list, related issues, and data collection methods (**Box 6**) used for the Viet Nam assessment.

Box 6. Table of Theme List and Potential Methods of Data Collection

Theme	Issues related to theme/topic	Proposed methods of data collection

Demographic profile of adolescents	Proportion of the total population; urban/rural differences
	Proportion in school at different ages in different regions
	Literacy, joblessness, marriage by age and sex
		Consulting secondary sources such as:
		  Census
		  Demographic and Health Surveys
		  Surveys by government or international organizations
		  Surveys by other organizations o research centres

Health status of adolescents	Morbidity and mortality of adolescents
	Identification of major causes of morbidity and mortality
	Reproductive health status of adolescents (pregnancy, abortion, STDs)
		As above, plus:
		  Annual reports by Ministry of Health
		  Provincial or district level records
		  Hospital/private clinic records

Adolescent health concerns	Adolescents' perceived health concerns and concepts of health Adolescent health concerns as perceived by others (health planners, youth leaders, teachers, health professionals)	Free listing, ratings, rankings Social mapping Focus group discussions In-depth interviews Secondary data Community meetings Key informant interviews
Content and nature of existing adolescent health policies and programmes	National health policies relevant to adolescents Rules and regulations affecting adolescent access and services (e.g. sexuality education, contraception, abortion) Adolescents as target cohort in national, provincial, district or village level policies and programmes	Health policies at various levels Relevant rules and regulations Documents outlining official health programmes (MOH, MOE) Documents outlining NGO programmes Community meetings Key informant interviews Observation

Adolescent health information needs	Perceived information needs of adolescents
	Adolescent information needs identified by others (health planners, youth leaders, teachers, health professionals)
		Above, plus:
		  Review of school and non-school health education programmes
		  Free listing, ratings, rankings
		  Community meeting
		  Key informant interviews

Step 4: Choosing methods

Box 6. Table of Theme List and Potential Methods of Data Collection (continued...)

Content, nature and use of existing health services for adolescents	Types of services at various levels Content of services (aims, human and fiscal resources, location) Services used by adolescents and usage patterns Perceptions of services and service needs by adolescents Service needs as perceived by others	Official health data, including usage patterns Review of content of services In-depth interviews Focus group discussions Observation
Health risks for adolescents	Population patterns of known risk behaviours, including "high-risk" groups Beliefs and perceptions about risks among adolescents themselves and others	Review of official health data at various levels Free listing, ratings, rankings Focus group discussions In-depth interviews Observation and mapping Community meetings Key informant interviews
Cultural, ethnic and geographic influences	Cultural beliefs, customs, language use influencing health risk and health-seeking behaviours (ethnic differences) Roles of family in health promotion (positive or negative) Impact of geographical factors (e.g. isolation, terrain, water quality and use, natural disasters) on risk and services	Review of census, DHS, other official data Review of relevant publications by other organizations Community meetings Key informant interviews Focus group discussions In-depth interviews Observation
Impact of economic status and employment	Absolute and relative poverty for various population cohorts Employment levels and wages for out-of-school youth Disposable income and spending patterns for youth in different environments Occupational health issues for adolescents	Review of DHS and other relevant reports Community meetings Key informant interviews Social mapping Focus group discussions In-depth interviews Observation

STEP 5: Constructing Topics for Free Listing, Check-lists and Question Guides

Now the Team is ready to move on to more concrete preparation for fieldwork. We need more than project objectives and preliminary theme list, although these documents serve as the starting point.

It is true that qualitative methods are flexible, use unstructured or semi-structured tools, and allow rich exploration of complex issues, giving an opportunity to reveal unexpected ideas. However, this does not mean that you should enter the field empty-handed.

Ethical guidelines should be followed, and Check-lists help ensure that informed consent is obtained and field data are properly stored to maintain confidentiality. Question Guides support you in interviews and discussions. If you invite adolescents to do free listing, you must be prepared with potential topics or questions to stimulate the activity.

Before going into the field, the Team should think about how and where free listing can be used. Look at the Theme List to decide which issues can be explored with this method.

There is no limit, in theory, to the number of topics that people can make lists about, so keep an open mind in the field. However, it is important to make a note of appropriate topics, and the wording you will use to ask participants to make lists.

Remember the basic objective of a needs assessment – to identify the gap between what exists and what is needed – and start with relevant topics. Topics may be different for different subgroups. Free listing can also be used with adults connected with the field of adolescent health. Examples follow **(Box 7)**, written in question format to prompt list-making. Be sure to pilot-test these.

Check-lists should include details so that Team members can keep track of data without breaching privacy or confidentiality. They will prompt for items such as researcher's name, date and time of interview, and selecting a code number that will be used on transcripts and stored separately from names or identifying details of participants. They should also ask for contextual information that will be used later to understand or explain results, and to make comparisons between individuals or groups.

>> **DECISION POINT**

Identify and pilot test topics or questions for free listing

Box 7. Topics for Free Listing (in question format)

For Adolescents	**For Health Professionals**
• What do you think are the main health concerns for people of your age?	• What do you see as the main health problems for adolescents in your area?
• What kinds of health information would you like to receive?	• What kind of information do adolescents want to have?
• Where would you like to obtain health information?	• What kinds of programmes would best meet the health needs of adolescents in your area?
• What kinds of health facilities would you like to have in your area?	
• What risky behaviours are practised by young people in this area?	

Such information may include, e.g. place of interview, age or school status of interviewees, number and sex of FGD members. Finally, check-lists summarize crucial components of informed consent procedures. Putting boxes next to each item helps to ensure these are not forgotten. Check-lists should be developed for observations, FGDs, in-depth interviews and key informant interviews, as set out below **(see Boxes 8-10)**. Except for observation, all methods require that you obtain informed consent.

Question Guides are sometimes called *interview schedules* or *topic guides*. Give careful consideration to the content and sequence of questioning or observation. Asking questions in the field will often be informal, and you will want to follow up statements to gain more information or a better understanding. The guide includes the main themes to be explored, and may contain possible questions, particularly when topics are sensitive or rely on knowledge of local terminology. Think about the order in which to raise different themes. If you try to conduct interviews or FGDs relying only on memory, you may forget to ask about important themes, spend too long on some at the expense of others, or struggle with awkward or sensitive topics.

Interviews and Focus Group Discussions (FGDs) normally start with a 'warm-up' phase to ensure that people feel comfortable and are willing to talk. Asking young people if they have a sporting hero may work well, but asking them if they have friends who use drugs will fail. Suggested questions are included in **Boxes 8-10**.

During this phase you can set the boundaries for FGDs: in particular, to explain that you want to hear from every participant, that there are no right or wrong answers, and that you want to hear their real opinions.

> **TIP**
>
> The 'warm-up' phase is the first step to successful interviews and discussions. If this is eliminated or rushed, you may not get good quality data later on. Remember, too, that useful data may also emerge from responses to 'warm-up' questions, so be sure to record the answers.

Some themes may be relevant for more than one type of field operation (e.g. during both FGDs and in-depth interviews with adolescents), while others are appropriate only for one. If you are using observation as a method, you should also prepare a guide that includes the issues you are interested in and particular items, behaviours, materials or patterns that you wish to observe.

Check-lists and Guides are only the beginning of the data collection process. Qualitative research relies upon spontaneous decisions about when to follow a particular line of questioning to obtain the information required.

Do not be satisfied with brief or simple answers, especially to key issues. Avoid question/answer, question/answer style. For FGDs, try to get the group discussing among themselves. For in-depth interviews, try to encourage lengthy, detailed replies.

Asking people for examples and stories can be effective. Don't stick blindly to the question guide. It is more important to collect good quality data than to 'finish' all the topics in the question guide.

Pilot-test the Check-lists and Guides to make sure that participants can understand your questions and that your order of questioning is appropriate. But you may find, even after piloting, that you need to modify these again in the field, especially as you meet a range of participants. This does not affect the validity of your research. Rapid assessments allow you to follow leads and be flexible, to gather diverse and unexpected information.

Over the next pages, we offer illustrations of Check-lists and Guides developed using the table **(Box 6)** formulated in Viet Nam and China. We include specific examples used for FGDs and in-depth interviews with adolescents, and interviews with key informants. Make your instruments in accordance with your objectives, themes and local conditions.

> **CAUTION**
>
> Question Guides are not Questionnaires! There is a risk that less experienced researchers may stick too closely to Question Guides or Topic Lists.
>
> The Team should discuss this danger before and during fieldwork to make sure that members understand the need for probing and follow-up questions, and the technique for doing so. See Part II for more detail on using specific methods.

>> **DECISION POINT** — *Develop and pilot-test lists and question guides for observation, FGDs and interviews*

Box 8. Example of an FGD Check-list and Question Guide for Adolescents

Check-list for FGD with adolescents

Names of facilitators, note-taker/s
....

Contextual information

This sheet will have confidential information identifying informants, and should be stored separately from all other data collected.

1. Identification number of FGD – this number should be used on all pages of notes and transcripts of this FGD
....

2. Who: number of participants, sex, school status, age, etc.
....
....
....

3. Where the FGD took place
....

4. When: date and time of FGD
....

5. Tape recorded? Yes/No

Check points

Researchers to give their names	☐
Briefly explain the purpose of the FGD	☐

<u>Ethical issues</u>

We will not use your name in our documents and your participation will be kept confidential.	☐
You may withdraw at any time. You do not have to answer every question.	☐
Are you willing to participate?	☐
Permission must be given if a tape recorder is being used	☐

Box 8. Example of an FGD Check-list and Question Guide for Adolescents (continued...)

Question Guide for FGD with adolescents

Remind participants that all opinions are welcome and valued.

Suggested 'warm ups':

    What sorts of activities do you do?

    How do you spend your time?

Suggested discussion topics:

1. **Health concerns** ☐
   - What are the major health concerns for young people of your age?
   - Do you think young people worry much about health in general?

2. **Health risks** ☐
   - What are the situations or activities around here that may be risky for young people?
   - What do you think is the best way to inform young people of health risks?
   - What do young people do in your area to avoid risk?

3. **Health services** ☐
   - Can you tell me something about local health services for young people?
   - If young people like you have a health problem, what do they usually do?
   - If you had a health problem would you be happy to go to the local health services?
   - Why or why not? (explore the barriers or good things about the health services)
   - If you were in charge of planning services for young people, what would you do?

4. **Health information needs and sources** ☐
   - Where do young people obtain information about health problems?
   - What kinds of health information would you like to have?
   - Where would you like to obtain such information, or not like to obtain it?

5. **Health promotion** ☐
   - What does being healthy mean to you?
   - What do young people here do to stay healthy?
   - How do you think society can help young people to stay healthy?

6. How important is health compared with other concerns of people your age? ☐

7. Other issues – summary of other issues you explored with this group of young people. ☐

Step 5: Constructing topics for free listings

Box 9. Example of a Check-list and Question Guide for In-depth Interviews with Adolescents

---

Check-list for in-depth interview with adolescents

Name of researcher...

Contextual information

This sheet will have confidential information identifying informants, and should be stored separately from all other data collected.

1. Identification number – this number should be used on all pages of notes and transcripts of this interview.
   ....

2. Who: name, age, sex, school status and other relevant circumstances
   ....
   ....
   ....

3. Where the interview took place
   ....

4. When: date and time of interview
   ....

Check points

Researcher to give his/her name ☐
Briefly explain the purpose of the interview ☐

<u>Ethical issues</u>

We will not use your name in our documents and your participation will be kept confidential. ☐
You may withdraw at any time. You do not have to answer every question. ☐
Are you willing to participate? ☐
Permission must be given if a tape recorder is being used ☐

Box 9. Example of a Check-list and Question Guide for In-depth Interviews with Adolescents (continued...)

Question Guide for in-depth interview with adolescents

Remind participants that all opinions are welcome and valued.
Suggested 'warm ups':
  How do you spend your time?
  Do you think boys and girls spend time in the same way?

Suggested discussion topics:
You will need to add more questions depending on results from free lists, the particular circumstances of the participant, issues that arise that need probing and the participant's responses. Make a record of any other issues that arise.

1. **Health concerns**
   - What are the major health concerns for young people of your age?
   - Do you think young people worry much about health in general?
2. **Health risks**
   - What are the situations or activities around here that may be risky for young people?
   - What do you think is the best way to inform young people of health risks?
   - What do young people do in your area to avoid risk?
3. **Health services**
   - Can you tell me something about local health services for young people?
   - If young people like you have a health problem, what do they usually do?
   - If you had a health problem would you be happy to go to the local health services?
   - Why or why not? (explore the barriers or good things about the health services)
4. **Health information needs and sources**
   - Where do young people obtain information about health problems?
   - What kinds of health information would you like to have?
   - Where would you like to obtain such information?
   - Are there some people or places where you would not like to obtain such information?
5. **Health promotion**
   - What does being healthy mean to you?
6. **Other issues**

Box 10. Example of a Check-list and Question Guide for Interviews with Key Informants

Check-list for in-depth interview with key informants
Name of interviewer..
Name of note-taker, if different..

Contextual information
This sheet will have the confidential identifying information of informants and should be stored separately from all other data collected.

1. Identification number—this number should be used on all pages of notes and transcripts of this interview.
....
2. Who: name and position of person interviewed ....
3. Where: organization of key informant and where the interview took place..
4. When: date and time of interview..
5. Tape recorder used? Yes/No

Check points Researcher to give his/her name ☐
Briefly explain the purpose of the visit ☐

<u>Ethical issues</u>
We will not use your name in our documents and your participation will be kept confidential. ☐
You may withdraw at any time. You do not have to answer every question. ☐
Are you willing to participate? ☐
Permission must be given if a tape recorder is being used ☐

Question Guide for in-depth interview with key informants
Add other questions depending on who is being interviewed. There will usually be many follow-up questions to elicit more detail, go deeper, clarify, etc.

1. Could you tell me something about your work here? ☐
2. What are your key responsibilities with regard to adolescents? ☐
3. What do you think are the major health concerns of adolescents? ☐
4. What has been done by your organization and other organizations to address these issues? ☐
5. What else do you think needs to be done? ☐
6. Other issues (record the other issues you explored with this particular key informant). ☐

STEP 6
Deciding on Sampling, Location and Responsibility

In planning rapid assessments, there is no rigid rule about which comes first: choosing methods, developing Question Guides, or deciding on sampling/location. Steps 4-6, therefore, may be undertaken in a different order from what is shown here, and even partly in tandem if there are sufficient numbers of skilled Team members.

Decisions taken in one step may lead to modification in another. This is a normal experience in planning for and conducting a rapid assessment. These plans are *tentative* and *flexible*, and can be altered in the field if necessary.

The quality of a rapid assessment depends in large part on appropriate selection of sample populations. These should be chosen with reference to your objectives and theme list. Ideally, samples would include numerous individuals and groups from diverse populations to enable a fuller exploration of themes and issues. However, this cannot be done rapidly, and is also very costly.

Purposive Sampling: non-random but strategic

The intent of a rapid needs assessment is to maximize opportunities to hear from people and groups most likely to be able to provide the data you are seeking. This can be accomplished by careful decisions to make best use of budgets and expertise.

Sampling should not be random, but *purposive*: that is, deliberately seeking individuals who can talk about the issues of interest. You will need to set some parameters, or selection criteria, to describe the type of people sought, and where you will seek them. Think carefully about different populations in your country, and identify which differences are important for meeting the objectives. Remember that you want to hear not only from young people, but from key informants.

Your Team should include members familiar with adolescent health concerns at national level, and thus able to offer informed guidance. It is also helpful to review a few appropriate health surveys or reports.

Aim for Diversity

In each country, there are **areas of diversity** among young people *(age, sex, school status, geographical location, social class, ethnicity, 'mainstream'/'high risk')*. 'High-risk' includes those involved in behaviours or lifestyles with potentially dangerous outcomes, such as unwanted pregnancy, transmission of STIs, drug addiction, occupational injury, or exploitation. At this point, the Team should discuss the following:

- Which differences are relevant?
- Where can these subgroups be located?

You may want to sample some adolescent girls in a poor mountainous region because this subgroup is likely to be influenced in behaviour and beliefs by isolation and economic pressures. You may also decide that it would be useful to meet adults who operate a youth hotline in the capital city.

Consciously try to identify people from diverse backgrounds, but make sure your primary focus is on the *groups of particular interest to your study*. In a national-level assessment, it would be a problem if your sample consisted primarily of 'at-risk' adolescents, because you would end up knowing little about the majority population. But it would also be a problem if you deliberately excluded 'at-risk' adolescents. Strive for balance, and be able to justify your choice of samples.

Box 11 offers some suggestions for sampling, but bear in mind the need to base decisions on demographic and geographic profiles of your country, as well as time and budget availability. *Strategic decisions based on a rational use of limited resources are crucial to the quality of the project.*

Box 11. General Suggestions on Sampling

Locations

URBAN AREAS. At least one. With a limited budget, it may be necessary to restrict this to the urban centre where the Team has its headquarters.

RURAL SITES. These should, if budget permits, include representation of your country's major regions. These may differ in terms of ethnicity, topography, economic activities, access to services and links to urban centres. In each site we suggest some specific locations:

1. Small town or market centre
2. Rural village (perhaps one hour from the small town)
3. More distant, marginal village

Samples

The YOUTH SAMPLE might include, for example:

1. Males and females of varying ages
2. In-school and out-of-school adolescents
3. Majority and minority ethnic groups
4. High-risk groups such as drug users, street children, workers in hazardous occupations

The KEY INFORMANT SAMPLE might include, for example:

1. Health care providers
2. Youth leaders
3. Members of NGOs working with street children

> **DECISION POINT**
> *Decisions about sample size, type and location, and areas of responsibility*

Which Comes First: Sampling or Method Choice?

It is clear that in making decisions about sampling, the Team is also making decisions about which specific methods it plans to use. This involves some back-and-forth movement, as the Team thinks about the most appropriate ways to hear from the target groups, and the cost (in time and money) of various methods. There will be limitations in whatever approach is taken, and these should be noted and debated.

A Fieldwork Plan

The Team should develop a fieldwork plan that details the location, type and number of each operation, assigns major responsibility for each, and estimates the time involved in every stage. If your Team is large enough, data gathering may happen simultaneously in more than one region.

The fieldwork plan should include:

- who does the work and where;
- age, sex, ethnicity, school status, etc. of adolescents interviewed;
- number of each field operation (e.g. 5 FGDs);
- type of key informants targeted;
- approach to recruiting participants;
- schedule of activities.

Here it may help to prepare two tables. The first summarizes planned field operations (locations, number of sites, specific methods and target samples). Be as concrete as possible. Please see **Box 12**, which illustrates a generic model.

The second table is a time line for the entire project. This shows target points for each stage of the assessment. Because several aspects happen simultaneously or continuously, it will provide a useful visual tool to identify work responsibilities and realistic expectations.

Naturally there is overlap between these two tables, which should be developed and used together. We offer an example of a fieldwork time line in **Box 13**. The time line will depend on the size of Team, budget and other expectations. Based on experiences in Viet Nam and China, we estimate that field data collection would take about three months.

Box 12. A Model of Planned Field Operations

Operations	Large Urban (3 sites)	Rural – less remote (3 sites)	High-risk group (e.g. street children) (3 sites)	Rural – more remote, e.g. mountainous (3 sites)	TOTAL
Key Informant interviews	5-10	5-10	5-10	5-10	20-40
Mapping, social mapping, observation	One mapping each by researchers and respondents (per site, as appropriate) Observation as indicated (1-2 per site)	One mapping each by researchers and respondents (per site, as appropriate) Observation as indicated (1-2 per site)	One mapping each by researchers and respondents (per site, as appropriate) Observation as indicated (1-2 per site)	One mapping each by researchers and respondents (per site, as appropriate) Observation as indicated (1-2 per site)	Approximately 20 mappings Approximately 12 observations
Focus Group Discussions	2 or 3 (1 Male, 1 Female, 1 Mixed)	2 or 3 (1 Male, 1 Female, 1 Mixed)	2 or 3 (1 Male, 1 Female, 1 Mixed)	2 or 3 (1 Male, 1 Female, 1 Mixed)	8 to 12
Free Listing	15-20	15-20	15-20	15-20	60-80 (if possible, have 2-3 topics)
Ratings from free lists	20 Females 20 Males	20 Females 20 Males	20 Females 20 Males	20 Females 20 Males	80 Females 80 Males
In-depth	10 Males 10 Females	10 Males 10 Females	10 Males 10 Females	10 Males 10 Females	40 Males 40 Females

Box 13. A Fieldwork Plan

ACTIVITY	Month 1				Month 2				Month 3			
	1	2	3	4	1	2	3	4	1	2	3	4
Make initial selection of research team, locations and target sample												
Travel to field and meet local officials, obtain permission, make further decisions about location of sites/samples												
Community meeting with local youth leaders, officials, relevant community organizations												
Train local adolescents to find sample for free listing, focus group discussion and in-depth interviews												
Mapping by researchers for familiarity and context												
Identify and interview key informants for each site												
Free lists with help from local adolescents												
Social mapping												
Focus group discussion at each site												
In-depth interview for each site												
Ratings of health by adolescents												
Collect secondary data on adolescent health needs												
Continue to refine "theme list"												
Continue to review progress, update notes (enter in computer if possible) and decide about sampling												

Step 6: Deciding on sampling

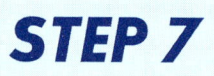

STEP 7
Entering the Field

After you have finished the fieldwork plan, consider the need for training or practice in methods for researchers, and make logistical decisions so the Team can enter the field quickly, smoothly and successfully. Effort now will save time and money and prevent field mistakes later.

Practise Unfamiliar Methods and Pilot-test Check-lists and Guides

It is ideal if ALL members have basic familiarity with ALL methods, as this will strengthen opportunities for triangulation and improve analysis of results.

In preparing for fieldwork in Viet Nam and China, the teams invited groups of youths to practise free listing and ratings, and group discussions. They also held central level Community Meetings, partly as practice.

If necessary, invite outside experts to discuss methods or act as facilitators in practice sessions. Trial the Check-lists and Question Guides (e.g. for FGDs or in-depth interviews), and modify these if necessary. Further modification of Question Guides may be necessary in the field.

Further Recruitment of Researchers

The Core Research Team may need to recruit additional research assistants for fieldwork, especially if several sites are being visited simultaneously. It is best if they come from a range of appropriate backgrounds.

Given the challenges of inter-generational communication, it may be wise to recruit young members, both male and female. On the other hand, research has shown that middle-aged women are most successful in talking to youths about sensitive topics.

While additional researchers need not be highly experienced, it is preferable for them to have some knowledge of qualitative research. They may need training and certainly should be monitored by the Core Research Team.

It is also highly recommended that local youths be invited to play a role in the project. They may help to recruit participants in the study (be sure they understand the selection criteria), identify key informants, and, where appropriate, conduct free-listing activities with youths. However, the Core Research Team should carefully monitor any research activities.

Permission to Enter the Field

The Core Research Team should write to or phone appropriate regional or local authorities to seek permission to conduct fieldwork. If telephoning, follow up with a written confirmation to avoid misunderstandings.

> **TIP**
>
> Be sure to seek permission well in advance of the field visit to avoid cancellations or changes. Be sure your fieldwork plans, and the project itself, are fully understood by local authorities to ensure smooth implementation.

Logistics and Materials

The Team will need to identify, arrange or purchase all material needed for the project. Check this against the fieldwork time lines and planned activities. Think about:

- transportation to, from and within field sites *(consider type needed, e.g. motorcycles or boats)*
- field accommodation *(so the Team will not be a burden for communities)*
- mobile phone, if appropriate
- pens, tape recorders, tapes, large paper, folders for storage of data, notebooks
- small gifts for participants *(e.g. pens used for free listing)*.

> **TIP**
>
> Consider whether there are special needs or problems in entering the field at certain times, such as holidays, harvest season, rainy season, etc.

STEP 8
Data Management and Analysis

The quality of your project and its findings will depend in large part on the skill applied to management and analysis of data. Some general suggestions are offered here, but these are not comprehensive.

Data Management

Implementing a rapid assessment always produces a large amount of paper, notes, transcripts, tapes, lists and maps.

There are several challenges in making sure these are kept safe and can be used fully in analysis. These include:

Confidentiality

- Use code numbers and store identifying information separately from transcripts or tapes, even during fieldwork.
- Be sure notes, transcripts, tapes, etc. cannot be easily accessed by non-researchers.

Safety and security of data

- All field records should be protected from accidents (e.g. leaking roof, damage by humans or animals).
- Computers and floppy discs can malfunction; make copies and store separately.

Planning ahead

- Write notes neatly and with enough detail to understand later on; draw pictures if this is helpful.
- A small spiral notebook for each researcher is essential for keeping records.
- Organize notes at the end of each day.
- Give ALL pages of transcripts and notes a code number to identify where each one originated.
- Leave a margin on notes and transcripts to make coding and organizing of data easier.
- Write only on one side of the paper for clarity and possible photocopying later.
- Test tapes and tape recorders before use.

Data Analysis

Different data collection methods use different types of analysis. For some, such as free listing, you will make tables that display lists, sorting or ratings (described in Part II). For secondary data, a summary, review or critique is appropriate.

Our focus here is on qualitative data analysis, which will comprise the bulk of your analysis work. Qualitative data are the words, sentences or observations noted in field records. The analysis involves identifying key concepts, themes and images that tell us meaningful things about the target community, and illuminating differences or similarities between diverse groups. Self-questioning, group debate, and working jointly on analysis can help guard against subjectivity.

Summary of recommended steps in analysis

- Good quality notes and transcripts are crucial. If possible, have a word-for-word record of what was actually said in interviews or FGDs (by transcribing the tape recording. When time does not permit, make notes as fully as possible, being sure you have collected some direct quotations.

- Read transcripts or notes several times.

- Look for 'key statements', i.e. ones that tell you something interesting or meaningful in relation to the research objectives and themes (remember, these may reveal some unexpected, new themes). Then highlight the 'key statements' with pens (or on computer).

- Number the original theme list.

- Using these numbers, code each 'key statement' in the margin. Some statements may relate to more than one theme, so you may need photocopies of notes.

- Decide how you want to organize the statements across the sample, and cut and paste (by hand or by computer) accordingly.

This step depends on what you are trying to analyse at that point, e.g. summary of views of rural out-of-school youth, a comparison of urban and rural out-of-school youth, etc. You will be guided partly by the original theme list and objectives, partly by what is known about demographics or health profiles in your country, and partly by the gradual emergence of insight and understanding that happens during qualitative research. You may also find it useful to present a Case Study in your report, so this step may focus on one individual or group.

- Discuss your findings and interpretations with other Team members. Open debate, and willingness to reflect, modify and re-interpret, are crucial to drawing sound conclusions from the data. The Team leader should actively seek a variety of views, but all opinions should be based on the evidence collected.

Investigators need to be constantly on guard against the danger of using evidence selectively to support their theories. . . . Scientific rigour can be maximized by careful checking that interpretations and conclusions are supported consistently by different strands of evidence. . . [through] triangulation (Campbell et al. 1999:61).

TIP

Seek external advice if your team does not feel confident about analysis. A list of helpful texts can be found in Appendix I.

STEP 9
Preparation of the Report

The final report should follow a standard research report outline, and cover study background, literature review, methods and rationale, findings and interpretations. It should summarize and synthesize key findings in view of the objectives. An overview of secondary data will be used to place your findings in context, and to discuss their implications. Limitations of methodology should also be discussed. Preliminary conclusions and recommendations should be included, with appropriate cautions. Below **(Box 14)**, we offer a guide to assist you in organizing the data systematically, and to serve as a reminder of the detail required for the report.

Box 14. Generic Guide for Preparation of Adolescent Health Needs Assessment Report

Note: *This guide follows the format ordinarily used in research reports and includes some detail describing the purpose and suggested content of each section. It is not meant to be rigid.*

Executive summary *(approximately 2-3 pages)* This section comes first and is an overview of the background and major findings, to gain familiarity prior to reading the report, or as a summary for those who will not read the entire document. It should include:

- Background to the assessment
- Research aims and objectives
- Data collection methods
- Sampling
- Data analysis methods
- Key findings and summary of recommendations

Table of contents Include all chapter headings and major subheadings, with page numbers.

Glossary Include all acronyms and terms that require explanation or definition. It is better to provide more, rather than fewer, definitions for the reader.

List of tables and figures List in order titles and page numbers of tables, figures and boxes. These may include, for example, demographic background of respondents, results of free listing, and summaries of secondary data. Consider offering visual variety, as well as recognizing the need for clarity.

Box 14. Generic Guide for Preparation of Adolescent Health Needs Assessment Report (continued...)

Chapter 1: Introduction

- Overview of project (project history, international interest in adolescent health, statement about the use of rapid assessment)
- Background to adolescent health in your country, demographic and epidemiological data of relevance (cohort size, morbidity and mortality, school retention rates, etc.)
- Research aims and objectives

Chapter 2: Methods

- Study design and rationale (population, methods of data collection and analysis)
- Ethical issues
- Limitations (e.g. time, budget, human resources, sampling bias, problems encountered, lack of generalizability)

Chapter 3: Findings/Results

Major findings in terms of study objectives belong here. Include details about what was learned from different populations (and secondary data), and how these relate to previous findings (if available). Presentation is important. The bulk of rapid assessment results will be explained in words. Free listing results can appear in numerical form (tables or graphs), but it is not appropriate to use statistical tests or probability calculations for rapid assessments.

Remember, you cannot present everything you learnt. A good, readable report will identify the most interesting and important findings, and describe these in a way that can be understood by others.

Organization is important. There are different options, each with advantages. Considering the variety of methods, participants and issues, it may be easiest to talk about each *study location*, summarizing key issues and differences/similarities between the sites. On the other hand, you may want to focus on *diversity in samples*, summarizing general findings in all sites (e.g., boys versus girls, older versus younger, in-school versus out-of-school). Or you could organize the report *by theme* to allow the identification of similarities and differences across different populations (including health providers or other key informants), in different locations, leading more logically to general conclusions relevant to future policy action.

Box 14. Generic Guide for Preparation of Adolescent Health Needs Assessment Report (continued...)

Lead the reader through your findings with brief introductory, summary or transition statements, and by using headings and subheadings. Words and observations are the data in qualitative methods, so use direct quotations (even if incomplete or ungrammatical) as illustrations.

Chapter 4: Discussion and recommendations

Discussion The discussion is the most important part of the report. Readers will want to know what your findings mean in the context of your country. Discuss key findings and their implications for programme or policy development. You may refer to previous projects or assessments, and comment on how yours compare or shed light on the issues. Be mindful of previous adolescent health activities. You may wish to consider the findings in terms of current trends in health, in your own social, economic, political and cultural context.

Recommendations These should briefly summarize the programmes, interventions, further study, or policy implications that follow logically from the assessment findings, remembering its objectives and limitations. They should be concrete and specific, and should indicate who should be responsible. The focus is likely to be on programmes and policies that can help fill the gap revealed by your rapid assessment. Specifically, consider:

- Which target groups for services, information or other interventions have been identified?
- What services are needed, where and by whom?
- What information needs have been identified?
- What policies would facilitate structures to enhance adolescent health and development?

Acknowledgements

Express appreciation for financial, technical or logistic support, and assistance from official or NGO leaders and participants in the study.

Reference list

Make a complete list following a standard, consistent format, of all publications or reports actually cited in the assessment report, including secondary data sources.

Summary: Guiding Principles for Undertaking Rapid Assessments

Rapid assessments are intended to collect as much data as possible in a short period of time. Therefore, there is always a risk that researchers may fail to make basic decisions appropriately because of a sense of being rushed. While some components can be done quickly, others should be done with care because of the central role they play in later stages of the assessment. A few reminders are offered here to help prevent such errors.

Avoid hasty decisions about topics and targets

Among the most crucial decisions are those relating to specific research topics, methods and target population. These cannot and should not be made at the outset of the project. Qualitative methods, which comprise the core techniques for rapid assessment, involve the gradual and **continuing emergence of** *themes* or issues of relevance to the study. This iterative process enables the discovery of concepts and issues identified by the population of interest, rather than those prescribed at the outset by the research team. Moreover, a basic understanding of the demographic and health indicators of the cohort is needed in order to select samples, which requires some preliminary review of secondary data.

Key issues for data collection

Certain considerations for the process of data collection can be seen as intrinsic to the philosophical assumptions and approach of rapid assessments. These include the following:

1. Develop a mechanism for feedback and *refinement of themes and approaches* in the field (e.g. evening round-table meetings) to challenge assumptions and stereotypes.

2. Use a wide *variety of methods* to strengthen the validity of findings.

3. Try to maximize the *participatory* potential of the project at all stages, because this is what sets rapid assessments apart from most other research approaches. Involving the community will facilitate the project, stimulate interest and sense of identification, enable researchers to benefit from local knowledge, and serve as a mechanism for dissemination of project findings. The 'community' includes young people, leaders, officials, key informants, and other relevant people.

4. Consciously set out to identify *diverse and contrasting* regions, populations, and sub-populations in order to explore the widest possible range of issues within the constraints of time, budgets and research experience. These contrasts include, but are not limited to the following:

   - Geographical (urban/rural; mountanous/lowland)
   - Age (younger/older)
   - Sex (male/female)
   - Ethnicity (majority/minority ethnic groups, if applicable)
   - Education level (lower/upper secondary; in-school/out-of-school)
   - Socioeconomic status (poor/middle-income/rich; working/unemployed; marginalized/'average')

Maximize skills, time and budget

Like all research projects, rapid assessments involve compromises. Invite open discussion to determine strengths and weaknesses of the Team, and apply this knowledge in determining locations, methods and field responsibilities. Not everything can be studied or known; concentrate on identifying what is most essential to your assessment, and seeking the most effective ways to investigate the issues.

Carefully plan time lines and itemize budgets. Seek to hear from those most likely to help you understand adolescent health needs, but be practical in allocating funds for hard-to-reach populations. Think laterally and creatively to supplement deficiencies by other means, and use triangulation to strengthen the validity of your interpretations and conclusions. Young people usually have a great deal of energy; try to make use of this in participatory methods and in widening the potential reach of the Research Team.

Finally, **good luck!** We are confident that you will find it enjoyable, stimulating and enlightening to listen to young people using these tools, and to learn more about adolescent health needs.

REFERENCES

Caldwell J.C., Caldwell P., Caldwell B.K. and Pieris I. The construction of adolescence in a changing world: implications for sexuality, reproduction and marriage. *Studies in Family Planning,* 1998, 29(2): 137-153.

Campbell O., Cleland J., Collumbien M. and Southwick K. *Social Science Methods for Research on Reproductive Health.* Special Programme of Research, Development and Research Training in Human Reproduction. Geneva, World Health Organization, 1999.

Dowsett G. and Aggleton P. Multi-site studies of the contextual factors affecting risk-related sexual behavior among young people in developing countries, 1997 (prepared for UNAIDS).

Efroymson D., Vu Pham Nguyen Thanh and Nguyen Quynh Trang. Confusions and contradictions: results of qualitative research on youth sexuality. In: Population Council and Ministry of Health, Youth Reproductive Health Seminar, 16 December 1997, Hanoi.

Michell L. and Amos A. Girls, pecking order and smoking. *Social Science and Medicine,* 1997, 44(12): 1861-1869.

UNFPA – United Nations Fund for Population Activities. *The State of World Population 1998.* New York, UNFPA, 1998.

WHO – World Health Organization. *Gender and Health: Technical Paper.* Women's health and development, Geneva, World Health Organization, 1998a.

WHO – World Health Organization. *Guidelines for Controlling and Monitoring the Tobacco Epidemic.* Geneva, World Health Organization, 1998b.

WHO – World Health Organization. *Programming for Adolescent Health and Development.* Report of WHO/UNFPA/UNICEF Study Group on Programming for Adolescent Health, WHO Technical Report Series 886, Geneva, World Health Organization, 1999.

PART II

AN OVERVIEW OF RAPID ASSESSMENT METHODS: WHAT THEY ARE AND HOW TO USE THEM

Introduction to Part II

Rapid assessments are conducted in a relatively short period of time, and it is not possible to use conventional survey methods to collect statistically valid information – nor is this the goal of rapid assessments. Instead, rapid assessments aim to gather rich, detailed information from diverse samples to gain a quick overview of issues and perspectives, ordinarily for the purposes of health programme development or evaluation.

Selection of methods for rapid assessments should be determined mainly by:

- research objectives and theme list, and
- budget, research expertise and time-frame.

Each method has benefits and limitations; the challenge in a rapid assessment is to make strategic decisions to maximize outcome.

The methods covered here include conventional qualititive tools, as well as some participatory techniques. Participatory techniques are often time-consuming, but create a sense of ownership of the project and outcomes. The value of the participation of local youth in the project cannot be overemphasized. This can help reduce the generation gap, foster good working relationships, and extend the amount of data collected in a short time-frame.

Part II offers a brief overview of data collection techniques most commonly used in rapid assessments. These will be presented in terms of their utilization for an adolescent health needs assessment. It is not intended as a comprehensive text for qualitative research methods. As noted in Part I, it is assumed that most members of the Core Research Team will have experience with qualitative research, if not with all the methods used in rapid assessments.

Appendix I provides further reference texts for qualitative research and rapid assessment techniques. We strongly recommend that you refer to these texts, or to others that cover use of methods and data analysis in greater detail.

For each method discussed, we cover the following aspects:

- role and objectives;
- sampling or sources; and
- limitations.

Each method fulfils a different purpose in the assessment, although there is overlap between some. In Part II we will provide information about the potential role for each method, as well as its limitations, to assist you in making your selection.

Some tips on conducting interviews and discussions

A primary objective of this assessment is to disover the perspectives of young people, and of those involved with adolescents. As a result, interviews and discussions will comprise a major and crucial part of data gathering efforts. We reiterate here that Question Guides should be used as starting points, and with flexibility. Richness, depth and meaning are revealed through a gradual process of probing and following-up by researchers, and through reflection by the research team. The art of interviewing and facilitating various research activities must be learnt and practised, but we would like to offer some pointers here **(Box 15)** that may act as helpful reminders. Additional suggestions will be made within individual sections.

Box 15. Tips for Interviews and Discussions

CAUTION	TRY TO
Don't be too formal or serious – it makes people nervous, and then they won't be open	Start with some warm-up questions to lighten the atmosphere and establish a rapport
Don't correct 'wrong' views Don't ask embarrassing questions Don't ask leading questions: • Do you know that smoking is dangerous? • Do you think it is acceptable for unmarried people to have sex?	Be open to new ways of thinking Ask neutral questions so that they can't guess your opinions: • *Do you think that smoking has any good or bad effects on health?* • *I have heard that some young people experiment with things like smoking, drugs or sex. Do you think these happen around here?*
Don't finish off a sentence or interrupt Don't jump quickly from topic to topic Don't summarize too quickly – you might not have heard the whole story	Probe and follow up to clarify and gather details: • *When you say adults never listen to adolescents, what do you mean?* • *Do you think other young people have the same feeling about adults?* • *Are there some adults who seem to listen better than others?* • *Can you give any examples of times when you felt an adult did listen to you?* Give appropriate verbal and non-verbal feedback *(nodding and looking interested can help)* Use simple, non-technical language Ask questions one at a time Be sure you understand what was said

Review of Secondary Data

We have already referred to the need for secondary data review within the adolescent health needs assessment. Because of the importance of this activity, we include further details on conducting the review here.

Role and Objectives

- To identify target adolescent population and issues (in terms of demographics and epidemiology)

- As another data source to lend validity to findings (through triangulation)

- In preparing the final report (as a data source, and for providing context for background and discussion)

Possible Sources of Relevant Secondary Data

Some data will be available from existing sources, e.g. census reports, departmental reports, NGO reports, health records, and other published and unpublished data from local and international sources, including the Internet. It may also be useful to review youth magazines or youth 'help' newspaper columns, if these exist, for further insights into what adolescents are being told, and what they are asking about in the popular press.

Limitations of Secondary Data Review

Not all secondary data are of equal relevance or validity. Some are out of date or based on flawed methods or sampling. It is important to consider potential weaknesses prior to using such data in the rapid assessment or final report. We offer below, in **Box 16**, a generic guide and checklist to assist in collecting, reviewing and assessing the relevance of these data.

CAUTION

Remember that secondary data need to be assessed for their limitations. Be sure to note the particular aims and methods of data collection, sampling techniques and methods of analysis. This helps in interpretation of the data and assessment of its relevance to the rapid assessment.

Box 16. Secondary Data Review and Check-list

Types of secondary data and possible sources

1. **Demographic information on adolescents**

   - Adolescent proportion of total population, rural/urban differences, gender differences *(demographic and other surveys by government and international agencies, NGOs and research centres)*
   - Literacy and schooling levels *(education department records, government and NGO surveys)*
   - Employment *(government and NGO records, employer records, occupational health surveys)*

2. **Health information**

   - Health status of adolescents *(hospital morbidity and mortality records, health surveys, private clinic records)*
   - Abortion rates and sexual and reproductive health issues *(maternal health records, family planning service records, NGO suveys, sex worker surveys, STI service records)*
   - Utilization of existing services *(service records)*

3. **Significant adolescent-related issues**

   - Adolescent concerns *(records from adolescent services, review of adolescent magazines and newspapers, surveys)*
   - Drug, tobacco and alcohol use *(epidemiological surveys, police records, NGO and support service records)*
   - Injuries and self-harm *(hospital morbidity and mortality records, police records for crashes, occupational health survey, rehabilitation records, suicide reports, mental health surveys)*

4. **Adolescent health policy**

   - National policy relevant to adolescents *(health policy documents at various levels, documents related to official programmes, documents outlining NGO programmes)*

Locating the sources

Government departments; government printing offices; head offices of international or local U.N. agencies or nongovernmental agencies; university departments (especially health, sociology); health service providers (curative and preventive services); youth magazines and other media; organizers of youth 'hotlines.'

Check-list for sources

- Record full bibliographic details (author, title, journal or book title, date, publishing information)
- The aims and objectives of the study
- The sampling strategy and data collection methods
- Biases and limitations of the findings
- Funding, reasons for study (agendas and stakeholders)

Community Meetings

Community meetings (CMs) are more than a data collection method; they are also a mechanism for securing support, identifying key informants and refining the theme list. Both roles are relevant for an adolescent health rapid assessment.

Community meetings are structured gatherings, organized by the research team, to which are invited stakeholders (those who play key decision-making roles in adolescent health) and gatekeepers (those who can enable, or prevent, access to target communities).

Community meetings are generally the first activity undertaken at each level (central, district, and, if appropriate, village) when implementing the rapid assessment. At these meetings, participants are informed about the project, its objectives and activities, invited to offer advice and secondary data, and asked for assistance in various ways to facilitate the project (e.g. generating new themes, providing local context, identifying relevant organizations and activities, locating samples, etc.).

Below **(Box 18)** we offer some other suggestions about organizing community meetings. Planning is important to ensure the right people are invited, the meeting goes smoothly, and that maximum value is obtained, so we have included a generic check-list and some ideas for discussion topics.

Role and objectives

- Expanding the theme list, and learning important details about local contexts
- Identifying Key Informants for later interviews
- Seeking logistical support and facilitation for fieldwork
- Preventing misunderstandings or anxieties that may hinder the project

In one sense, community meetings have both an open and a hidden agenda. For the open agenda, community meetings are important sources of data and contacts, as well as opportunities for rapid familiarization with important issues and structures. They can also serve as a reference group for dissemination of your findings. For the hidden agenda, community meetings can help reassure stakeholders and gatekeepers that you value their input and expertise and will not act as trouble-makers.

CAUTION

When inviting participants to a community meeting, it is best to call it simply a "meeting", otherwise there may be confusion over terminology and purpose.

Who should be invited to the Meeting?

Use your networks, existing data, or local knowledge to draw up invitation lists. It is likely that you would invite responsible government authorities, leaders in youth organizations, health programme managers and planners, health providers, principals and teachers, and leaders of NGOs working with youth (including high-risk populations).

There is no definite number you should invite, but try to include all relevant people, and those whom it is diplomatic to include. **Box 17**, opposite, is the invitation list used in Ho Chi Minh City, headquarters of the Core Research Team in Viet Nam. Community meetings were also held at district level during field implementation of the assessment.

Planning the Meeting

After preparing the invitation list, decide on venue and timing, and write an invitation letter, sending it out well in advance. Be sure the venue is appropriate in terms of size, location and facilities. Think about dividing into smaller groups for discussion, privacy, lighting, refreshments and comfort. In some countries it may be appropriate to reimburse transport expenses.

Decide beforehand who will chair the meeting, what you will say about the project, who will facilitate small groups (you may wish to use participants), and what topics to discuss. Some of these details may be included in your invitation letter to stimulate reflection prior to the meeting. We have summarized key points that may be useful for planning in **Box 18**.

Box 17. Community Meeting Invitation List Used at Team Headquarters in Viet Nam

- Officials from the Health Department of Ho Chi Minh City
- Managers of city primary health care programmes, including child health and reproductive health services
- Clinicians providing reproductive health services to adolescents
- Members of the Viet Nam Youth Union and Women's Union
- Lecturers and researchers from universities and medical schools
- Officials from the Education and Training Department
- Clinicians from the mental health centre
- Local television and newspaper reporters
- Officials from the Committee for Protection and Care of Children

(Total number attending was approximately 25)

Limitations of community meetings

Community Meetings cannot replace in-depth, individualized approaches. Participants may not feel free to speak openly about sensitive topics, especially if these are controversial. Also, discussion may be dominated by participants with strong personalities or high-ranking positions. Finally, as in all group discussions, skill is needed to ensure it is managed well. This is a greater challenge when influential people are part of the group. Hence, a strong chairman is an advantage.

Box 18. Check-list for Community Meetings

Identify an appropriate time and venue for the meeting; consider space requirements (including for small group discussion), audiovisual needs, privacy from intrusion, comfort and access to refreshments. ☐

Send invitation from appropriate person in timely fashion, covering: ☐
- Brief overview of the Rapid Assessment project
- Acknowledgement of need to learn from existing projects and expertise in a group meeting
- Venue, date, time of meeting

Make decisions about responsibility for arranging materials, rooms, refreshments, welcoming, feedback sessions and thank you. ☐

Plan the meeting. ☐
One possible format is:
- Welcome by appropriate person and thanks to participants for coming
- Briefly introduce the project and Core Research Team
- Explain purpose of Rapid Assessment for Adolescent Health Needs
- Invite sharing of information (including reports, data) and expertise to assist the Team in efforts to investigate important issues
- Suggest breaking into groups of 6-10 people to discuss questions, e.g.:
  1. *What are the key health concerns for adolescents in your location?*
  2. *What has been done to address these health concerns?*
  3. *What needs to be done in the future?*
- Synthesize findings and thank participants for attending (provide refreshments)

After the meeting, collate findings, discuss relevance to the project, identify potential Key Informants and gatekeepers and maintain contact details for later communication. Follow up with a letter to participants with a summary of the key points. ☐

Key Informant Interviews

Although the rapid assessment will focus primarily on the perspectives and experiences of adolescents, non-adolescent 'key informants' can provide detailed information and special expertise. They can also reveal the attitudes of adults towards young people.

Key informants may be stakeholders or gatekeepers in adolescent health, or they may have no particular position or authority. For example, a known drug distributor is an ideal key informant on drug sales; a policeman is not. A religious leader is ideal to explore religious opinions about sex education or HIV/AIDS prevention advice, but not about young people's sexual practices. Choosing key informants depends on what you want to know. They are most useful in providing information not available from published sources.

Key informant interviews are usually semi-structured interviews, and should be conducted in person. Although you will draw up a list of potential informants, don't forget that you may meet one opportunistically, and these informal interactions can yield useful data.

Role and objectives

- To provide background information useful for refining the theme list or identifying target populations
- To supplement secondary data about adolescent health and health risks
- To hear about experiences working with adolescents
- To shed light on the attitudes of those involved in adolescent health

Choosing key informants

It may be helpful to think of this sample in terms of who knows a lot and who will talk about important topics in the assessment. Try to find people who may have different perspectives on the same issue, or who are located in different places. These might be, e.g. an official from the Ministry of Education who has developed a school health programme, a teacher who uses the curriculum, and a member of a community organization that supports young people in difficulties. Others might be police or shopkeepers where adolescents congregate.

Locating key informants may take some time and networking, because many of those who work with adolescents also have other responsibilities. Use existing contacts, the Community Meeting and field activities. The following list may be helpful in starting to identify key informants for your assessment:

- Health personnel, particularly those with responsibilities for adolescent health, reproductive health, or other focus on older children

- Government organizations responsible for adolescent health

- School health personnel

- Staff at UNICEF, Population Council and other international agencies that may have programmes and information concerning adolescent health issues

- NGOs with programmes in potential target areas

Key informants in major urban centres can often direct researchers to persons in local communities who can be of assistance in the data collection at the grassroots level.

Preparation for interviews

You should be well prepared for a key informant interview. A Check-list and Question Guide (see example, **Box 10**, in Part I) will ensure that all important questions are covered, and that you have explained about confidentiality and anonymity.

CAUTION

In some places, asking for an 'interview' may create suspicion, anxiety or self-consciousness. It may be better to ask simply for a chance to meet the informant to talk about adolescent health issues, and avoid the word 'interview' altogether.

As in all semi-structured interviews, follow-up, probing questions are essential for revealing important details. Key informants may have to be contacted more than once in the course of data collection, and thus become valuable advisers. Developing a good rapport with key informants is essential.

There are two main options for recording data from key informant interviews. Taking notes emphasizes that what he or she has to say is considered important. However, if you cannot write fast enough to record the details, you may need to use a tape recorder, but be mindful of the self-consciousness this may produce, and the limitations of fallible technology. Whichever option you choose, seek permission from the informant and assure them of the confidentiality of the information.

TIP

Be sure to carry your notebook at all times in the field to make notes during or after any chance meetings with key informants. For example, researchers in Viet Nam found themselves unexpectedly spending 10 minutes with the director of a local health centre, who was happy to discuss adolescent issues as she transported the team to a local school to meet adolescents.

Limitations of key informant interviews

Information that you obtain from key informants will be limited by your access to them (they may be busy and unable to meet you, or only able to meet you briefly). Some degree of skill is needed to interview effectively, especially if informants are nervous or suspicious. Furthermore, they may be unwilling to disclose sensitive information, or to speak truthfully, because of their position in the community, despite being assured of privacy and confidentiality. Remember that what you hear may not be accurate, either due to the wrong choice of informant, or because they are influenced by personal prejudices or a desire to gain professional advantage.

Focus Group Discussions

Focus group discussions (FGDs) are group discussions on a particular topic, led by a facilitator, and used for obtaining information about people's attitudes and beliefs. The technique relies on the group dynamic. FGDs can supplement initial key informant interviewing and mapping activities (described later), and are often helpful in the early phases of data collection to solicit a wide range of ideas. It is important to remember that FGDs are a group process, not a set of individual interactions.

Role and objectives

- To investigate beliefs, attitudes and concepts of behaviour quickly and economically
- To gather exploratory data, such as locally used terms, or local patterns of behaviour
- To have direct communication with a population, literate or not
- To explore ideas building on group responses
- To obtain feedback on proposed or existing services

During an FGD a facilitator uses a loose Question Guide to stimulate discussion. Ordinarily, FGDs are tape-recorded to take full advantage of the wealth of information offered. However, transcribing these takes many hours. In rapid assessments, note takers, who strive to write down all important points in the language actually used, are often utilized instead. Audiotapes can provide a backup for checking notes, but *ask permission before taping*.

Sampling issues

- Purposive, non-random sampling is used. You must select participants who know something about the topic, have an interest in it, and can speak from a variety of perspectives. They do not 'represent' the wider population, nor reveal prevalence of views, but that is not the purpose of FGDs.

- Participants should feel comfortable with each other. Homogeneous groups usually work best because discussion is not inhibited by power differences (e.g. between young and old), or shyness between the sexes. If possible, have separate FGDs for younger and older adolescents, for boys and girls, and for those of very different educational or social levels.

Pointers for conducting FGDs

- Think about preparation.

    Using the theme list, plan what you want to ask about and construct a Question Guide to help you to remember important topics. This is a loose guide, and should be used flexibly as a starting point, to be followed by additional questions to seek responses from all participants. Make a Check-list of important logistic and ethical points. Examples of Check-lists and Question Guides are found in Part I under Step 5.

- Size of the FGD.

    FGDs usually involve 6 to 10 participants. Larger groups are difficult to run and control; smaller groups may be stiff and also lack diversity of views.

- Venue is important.

    The venue should make participants feel secure and relaxed. For example, holding an FGD with sex workers at the Health Department may not encourage them to speak freely. The place should be quiet so that tape recording (if used) is clear, and so participants can hear each other.

- Clarity about the process is important.

    Let participants know in advance the general purpose of the discussion. When it starts the facilitator and note taker should introduce themselves, and reassure participants about confidentiality, seeking permission for tape recording. Tell them there are no 'right' or 'wrong' answers, and that you wish to hear from everyone. Emphasize that there may be many points of view, and they are encouraged to express their own, but that they are under no obligation to talk about any subjects they wish to avoid.

- Asking questions and using the Guide.

    After asking some 'warm-up' questions, the facilitator should collect basic demographic information about participants to provide context. Then raise the main issues of interest, gradually moving from one to another. Be open to new themes at every point, as you may hear quite unexpected ideas.

- Preventing discomfort or embarrassment.

    Participants should not be encouraged to talk about their own personal details and confidential information should not be raised. The facilitator must ensure that individuals are not humiliated or singled out for criticism in the FGD. Sometimes 'narrative' FGDs are used. These allow the facilitator to describe fictitious characters or hypothetical situations to seek responses without personal implication. For single-sex FGDs it is advisable that facilitators and note takers are the same sex as participants.

- Tact and skill are needed for FGD management.

    All participants should be encouraged to speak, with special attention to encouraging shy members, or to resolving smoothly problems that arise where people are domineering, negative or interrupting **(see Box 19)**.

It is usual to summarize main discussion points at the end of an FGD, highlighting areas of agreement and disagreement, so that participants can clarify or add extra information. Remember to thank them for participating, and to offer refreshments, during which informal discussion may continue.

- Data management should begin as soon as possible.

As soon as possible after each FGD, the facilitator and note taker should discuss the process, and expand notes. For a one-hour FGD the note takers may need two hours to do this properly. Verbatim quotes should appear in the expanded notes. Also, key local expressions should be listed. If hand-written notes are the main record, you may wish to listen to tapes, if available, to improve the quality of the transcript.

Limitations of FGDs

- Not a natural setting *(unlike observation)*
- Researcher has less control over data to be generated because of group dynamics
- May be biased by dominant members
- Some find the group setting inhibiting, *especially if the topic is sensitive*
- Much depends on skill of facilitator
- Context is critical to interpret data

Box 19. Managing 'Difficult' FGD Participants

Problem	Tips for Managing
Dominant Participant May be a youth leader and knowledgeable, but tries to answer every question immediately, making others feel less confident and reluctant to speak.	Avoid contact with the participant. When the participant begins speaking, politely say, *Your points are very interesting, but we haven't heard anything yet from some of the others.*
Quiet Participant Does not speak spontaneously, and, even when invited, may simply say, *I don't have any idea about the topic,* or, *I feel the same way as the last speaker.*	Remember to mention at the start of the FGD that the objective is to hear from everyone. You can try to address questions directly to the Quiet Participant by name, but don't force him/her to speak – it is embarrassing.
Interrupting Participant Keeps interrupting others and interfering with the natural flow of discussion.	Listen briefly, then say politely, *I do want to hear from you, but I think the other participant hadn't finished speaking.*
Negative Participant Speaks with hostility or aggression to you or others in the FGD.	Be careful not to anger this participant further, or to create divisions in the FGD. Try not to be defensive – it is unlikely that the Negative Participant is targeting you. Listen, stay calm, and invite others to offer their opinion (peer pressure may be an effective tool).

Adapted from Agyepong I. Aryee B. Dzikunu H. and Manderson L. *The Malaria Manual*. Methods for Social Research in Tropical Diseases No. 2. UNDP/World Bank/WHO Special Programme for Research and Training in Tropical Diseases, Geneva, World Health Organization, 1995, p.39.

In-depth Interviews

In-depth interviews are two-way managed conversations used to reveal attitudes and perspectives about a topic. In-depth interviews are different each time because the direction of discussion stems from the unique responses of each interviewee. Question Guides help the interviewer maintain focus and cover key issues, but are only starting points.

Role and objectives

- To explore in detail the concepts, beliefs and attitudes of individuals

- To discuss issues that may be too sensitive for FGDs

- Respondents are not forced to choose from a predetermined list of answers to fixed questions, but can answer spontaneously, thus encouraging the emergence of unexpected themes and issues

Using in-depth interviews for 'case studies' for rapid assessments

In-depth interviews can often be very lengthy. For a rapid assessment, you may wish to limit these to just a few cases to illustrate important adolescent health issues. These might include, for example, an unmarried young mother, a young man doing dangerous work, or a youth activist who works with adolescents. The data can then be presented as case studies, with identifying information changed to ensure confidentiality.

Case studies might cover detailed information about risk behaviours and concepts of risk, health-seeking behaviours, or other relevant issues. Case studies may be based on interviews alone or supplemented by observation and documentation.

The number of case studies collected depends very much on the timetable of the project and available resources. If there are adequate field interviewers available, it is desirable to have 10 to 15 cases from each major category of adolescent (according to the key areas of diversity identified by your Team). This will allow for individual variation, as well as similarities and differences across groups (or locations).

Sampling issues

- Purposive, directed by objectives and theme list (not random)

- Might include:

    ○ extreme cases (adolescents at extreme risk, e.g. street children)

- ⌑ homogeneous cases in different locations (e.g. young, out-of-school boys)
- ⌑ 'typical' cases (to represent different types of youths)
- ⌑ 'politically' important cases (those who can speak on behalf of influential groups)

- Located by using contacts developed during Community Meetings, key informant interviews and FDGs.

Pointers for conducting in-depth interviews

- Think about preparation.

  Use the theme list to construct a Question Guide to help you to remember important topics. This is a loose guide, to be used flexibly as a starting point, and followed by additional questions to go deeper. Make a Check-list of important logistic and ethical points. Examples of these are found in Part I, under Step 5.

- Setting and atmosphere are important.

  These should be appropriate to the person and the topic. The way you dress and speak can either increase or minimize real or perceived differences (e.g. social class, age, culture or sex). It is a good idea for researchers to be the same sex as interviewees. Arrange a place that offers comfort and privacy, bearing in mind the need to maintain an appropriate distance between researchers and those who are not yet legal adults. A local youth leader may be able to suggest a venue, which may be in a health centre, school, coffee shop or community centre. Try to keep interruptions to a minimum.

- Clarity about the process is important.

  Let the interviewee know in advance the general purpose of the interview. On the day, introduce yourself (and a note taker, if relevant), explain about voluntariness and confidentiality, and seek permission if you are using a tape recorder. Note that there are no 'right' or 'wrong' answers, that you wish to hear his/her own opinions.

- Using the Guide.

  After asking some 'warm-up' questions, the researcher may decide first to collect basic demographic information (e.g. age, school status), or instead, go directly to the main issues of interest, gradually moving from one to another. While it is common to start with easy-to-answer demographic questions, sometimes these seem too direct or even embarrassing, while those based on the themes seem less confronting. Be flexible in the field. The main thing is to be open to new themes and issues at every point, as you may hear quite unexpected ideas.

- Preventing discomfort or embarrassment.

  Watch carefully for any signs of distress or embarrassment. Youths may initially be shy about talking to a stranger, but you should be able to recognize any strong negative reactions, which could be linked to personal circumstances, memories or religious sensitivities. Be ready to change the subject or, if necessary, refer the interviewee to an appropriate person for support or advice. Narrative interviews, in which the researcher describes fictitious characters or hypothetical situations, can be used to seek responses.

- Tact and skill are needed to draw out discussion.

  Establishing a rapport and a relaxed environment are crucial to collecting good quality data. Be patient, as many young people take some time to feel at ease with adult strangers. Try to show genuine interest through comments and body language to help youths feel confident that you will really listen. Try never to show shock or disapproval, which would quickly stop the flow of conversation.

  If adolescents are not talkative, it is tempting to ask a string of questions, one after the other. Try to avoid sounding like an interrogator! Asking people to describe actions or events often helps yield richer, fuller data.

  If you are trying to understand health-seeking behaviour, you might ask, e.g. *Can you tell me what you did the last time you got sick, how you managed to get well again?* Depending on the level of detail in the response, you may want to follow up with a few questions to help keep the talk going, e.g. *What advice did the pharmacist give you?* or *Do you think it's better to go to the pharmacist or to a doctor?* etc.

- Keeping a careful record.

  Because it takes many hours to transcribe one hour of recorded interview, it is better in a rapid assessment to use hand-written notes for interviews. These should contain all important comments, in the real words of the interviewee, if possible. During, or immediately after the interview, note any new themes that emerged, minor misunderstandings, topic avoidance, emotional reaction, your feelings about the interview, and describe the setting.

Limitations of in-depth interviewing

- Difficult to use with people who don't like speaking or who talk a lot but lose focus

- Analysis is more difficult and time-consuming than for standardized interviewing

- Interviewer must judge instantly whether or not to follow up unexpected topics

- Interviewer must take complete notes (or use a tape recorder) without disturbing the respondent.

Observation

Through observation we can document what people *actually do,* which may be different from what they say. This is a powerful tool for triangulation of data. Observation is something we all do naturally and constantly, but is underutilized as a data collection tool. By making observation structured and systematic, it is possible to obtain very rich and valuable data. There are two main types of observation: *obvious* (and reactive), and *unobtrusive* (and non-reactive).

In *obvious* reactive observation, people know they are being observed. They may then react to the observer's presence, and behave in a way they believe is expected or wanted by the observer, rather than naturally.

In *unobtrusive* observation, participants are unaware they are being observed and behave as they usually would. There can be serious ethical implications, however.

As a data collection tool, observation can be made systematic by creating lists of observable items that are of relevance to the study objectives and themes. For instance, we could identify relevant, observable aspects of behaviour of street youth: with whom do they interact, reactions to and by authorities, e.g. police, their 'hang-outs', what they do when they 'hang out', etc.

Role and objectives

- Can observe directly what people actually do
- See with 'fresh eye' aspects not visible to people living or working in the setting *(practices, habits, relationships, etc.)*
- Learn about behaviours too sensitive to talk about in interviews
- Understand how organizations operate and how people perform their functions
- For purposes of triangulation
- Explain context to aid interpretation

Sampling issues

- Purposive, non-random (select items, places and people you want to observe, based on the theme list and objectives)
- Decide if you want to observe similar things in different locations, or different things in one location, or some combination of these

- Make tentative decisions about duration of observation, but try to be flexible (and keep notes about what really happened).

- There may be opportunities for 'chance' observation of relevant items – always keep a notebook with you.

Pointers for conducting observations

- Make lists of observable items.

    Using the theme list, identify items that can be observed. These may be different in different locations.

- Prepare a Check-list and Question Guide.

    Your Check-list will cover items such as observer's name, place and date of observation, and whether it was obvious or unobtrusive. The Question Guide will cover the particular items or issues of interest. Include a category of "other" items, because you are likely to see unexpected items of interest.

- Decide on level of involvement and visibility.

    In a rapid assessment you can strive to be less obvious by, for example, sitting in a coffee shop where young people gather, or (for younger researchers) taking part in activities such as playing video games. Your level of visibility may influence both what you see, and how others behave. Think about whether you need to seek permission to conduct the observation.

- Field notes must be clear and complete.

    Describe what you observed, heard, and your thoughts about it. For example, if you were observing service provision in an STI centre used by adolescents, you

    might note the location of clinic, opening hours, waiting times, privacy, system of calling out names, sex and age of clients and clinicians, information posted on the wall or given to clients, whether or not drugs for treatment could be purchased there, and style of interactions between clients and providers (if visible).

Limitations of observation

- What you see on one occasion may be an exception, and not usual

- People may change their behaviour if they know they are being observed

- You may misinterpret what you see because you lack contextual information

CAUTION

Don't be too quick to draw conclusions about what you see, or don't see. For example, if young people aren't at a youth centre on a particular day, it may not mean they don't like it, but that they are busy with the harvest. Conversely, don't conclude that adolescents like a centre because it is crowded. It could be a special event drawing them, or even that there are no other places for young people to gather. Use observation to supplement other methods, and be tentative about your interpretations.

Mapping by Researchers

Mapping is carried out by researchers with the help of informants. It usually involves unstructured observations, often from walking through the study area, to become familiar with local conditions and customs, observing, e.g. the extent of poverty, time use, avenues for health education, etc.

Simple, hand-drawn maps can show locations of health providers, 'risk behaviour' (such as motorcycle racing), movements of persons such as street children, group hang-outs, loitering places, recreational areas, etc. Informal, unstructured interviews can be conducted at the same time. Mapping enables the researcher to get a 'feel for the community'.

Role and objectives

- Using informal sketches to make a visual record of relevant features of a community
- Gaining familiarity with important local context and situation for the research team
- Often used in combination with informal interviews.

Limitations of mapping by researchers

This tool does not produce data for analysis, but merely for background understanding. The usefulness of this tool will depend on the ease and accuracy with which researchers utilize it, as some people do not feel comfortable in making maps.

Social Mapping

In social mapping, the maps are drawn by community participants in order to develop rapport and participation. Usually social mapping is done by a group of five or more individuals. Social maps show how people perceive spatial arrangements of available facilities and important landmarks. For example, street children could be asked to draw where they go to earn money, sleep, eat, seek medical assistance, etc. Social maps also create a powerful tool for generating discussions about the specific activities identified on the maps.

Role and objectives

- To stimulate discussion between researchers and participants
- To understand the spatial view of adolescents
- To collect information about behaviours, activities and their relative locations

Sampling issues

Social mapping within the rapid assessment is likely to be done by groups of adolescents. As it is usually not undertaken as a separate tool, but as part of a discussion, the sampling issues relative to FGDs should be considered here.

Pointers for using social mapping

- Preparation is important.

    Think about the situations or activities that can be drawn by adolescents. Decide how you will describe what you want them to do, because there may be confusion, awkwardness or uncertainty at the outset. Specific questions can stimulate map drawing. Provide large paper and have enough to make a second or third start. Pencil is not very bright, but has the advantage of being erasable. Coloured marker pens are more fun to use and produce a livelier outcome. Be sure you have space to draw, either on the floor, table or wall. If possible, provide simple refreshments and small gifts (e.g. drawing pens).

- Explain the process clearly.

    Introduce yourselves and explain the purpose of the assessment, and the content of each activity (e.g. mapping and FGD) and likely time-frame. Divide them, if necessary, into smaller groups, and ask them to choose someone to do the drawing, explaining that the others will contribute ideas.

- Use the final product

    Hang the map up (be prepared with tape), and invite the group to talk through interesting things on the map. Participants are likely to have plenty to say, much to debate, and many things to laugh about as they see a visual outline of part of their world.

Limitations of social mapping

Social mapping does not work equally well with all populations and issues. Some people may perceive it as a childish activity, while others may feel too shy to draw. Thus, it is important to clarify why you want to use the tool, and whether it will reveal the information you are seeking. It may be more difficult for inexperienced researchers to facilitate the map making, as well as to use it as a discussion tool. Practice is recommended in using this activity.

Free Listing

Free listing is a powerful, underutilized tool for rapidly gaining information. The technique is simple: the researcher asks participants to generate a list of items that come to mind in response to specific questions. In a rapid assessment, free lists from 15-20 informants in each location are usually adequate, but they are cheap and easy to collect, and there are benefits in getting more.

A series of lists provides a useful inventory. If we collect a list of health problems from only one person, we may get 6 or 8 items (problems). When we collect 15 lists we are likely to get 20-40. Lists also give valuable added information about the salience* of individual items which can be calculated easily. Additional activities to maximize data gathering with this tool will also be described.

Role and objectives

- Identifying concepts, attitudes and practices related to topics from different types of individuals
- A rapid, cheap tool useful for expanding knowledge
- Can be written or dictated, if illiterate (good way to learn from shy adolescents)
- Useful for stimulating group discussion for deeper exploration of issues

Sampling issues

Purposive, non-random methods are used to identify samples from different demographic backgrounds. Youth associations, technical training centres and schools may be able to help locate samples, but it is important to hear from those who may be more difficult to find. Word-of-mouth and snowball sampling can be useful.

Make sure the selection criteria are clearly explained if others are assisting, or you may not get the types of people you are expecting. Also, although it is easy to collect many lists, keeping track of lots of paper is not so easy.

---

* Salience simply refers to the extent that any topic is on people's minds. For example, if we ask people to tell us all their current problems, "lack of money" is likely to be mentioned frequently.

Pointers for free listing

- Prepare topics and questions.

  Examine the theme list and related issues to identify topics that are appropriate for free listing. For example, adolescents may find it easy to make lists of risky behaviours, or specific health information they would like to have. But they may be able to mention just one or two items if you ask them to list adolescent health programmes in their community. Decide how many lists you will seek from each person, and the exact wording for each question (you may need to ask a local informant for terminology or context).

  There are many kinds of lists that can contribute to the assessment, depending on age, sex, social class or geographical setting. These may include:

  1. The main health concerns of adolescents in your area
  2. What do adolescents around here do to protect their health (to stay healthy)?
  3. What are the programmes/activities you think would help make you more healthy?
  4. What are the main health risks in this area for young people?
  5. What are the dangers of tobacco use?
  6. List the places where you would like to obtain health information.
  7. What kinds of health information would adolescents like to have?
  8. Who do you talk to about puberty?

- Prepare for the activity.

  Choose a time and place that are convenient for participants, and invite them in advance. Think about whether you want to divide the group by sex or age. This is more relevant if you plan to hold an FGD with participants.

  Explain the activity, emphasizing that there are no right or wrong responses, and that they should write the first things that come into their minds. Stress that lists may be of different lengths, because each person has individual ideas or concerns. Put either a time limit (e.g. five minutes) or a number limit (e.g. no more than 10-15 items), because otherwise the lists may be too long to summarize rapidly, or participants may feel bound to keep adding items just to fill in time.

  Make sure there is space to write privately, enough paper and pencils/pens. It may be helpful to write the question on a big sheet of paper as a reminder, especially if they are making more than one list. You can use the same paper for displaying the results, including salience, to prompt discussion.

  If funds permit, offer light refreshments and a small gift (e.g. pens used to write lists) as a thank you.

Limitations of free listing

Compared with FGDs or in-depth interviews, free listing offers less depth and fewer layers of complexity. With many cards and individuals using these, free listing can be a challenge. There is also the danger of misunderstanding terminology or intent of some items, especially if these are abbreviated or written unclearly. Follow up with some individual or group discussion to arrive at a shared understanding of the listed items.

Pile Sorting

Pile sorts enable items obtained from a free list to be ranked in order (for instance, in order of priority to the community) or rated on a predetermined scale. This provides deeper understanding of perceptions, and gives the community a voice in determining priorities. Salience* tells us only how often an item is mentioned, but may not reflect its importance. Pile sorting can also be used to show linkages between items, thus revealing beliefs and concepts useful for health planning.

Role and objectives

- Understand the relative importance to individuals/communities of free-listed items
- Reveal views through grouping of topics

The most common types of pile sorting are Rating and Grouping. Tips on conducting these activities are described below.

Pile Sorting: (1) Conducting a Rating Exercise

1. Select 20-25 health concerns from those items most commonly mentioned (most salient). You may also supplement these with others that interest the research team.

2. Write each item on a separate card in the local language.

3. Number the cards (on the reverse side).

4. With all the cards spread out (on a table or the floor), ask the group to identify two that are considered the most dangerous, and another two that are considered least serious.

5. Place the selected cards at two different ends of the table, one end representing the most serious and the other the least serious.

6. Ask participants to sort the remaining cards between these two piles (any remaining ones can then be classified as 'intermediate').

---

* Salience simply refers to the extent that any topic is on people's minds. For example, if we ask people to tell us all their current problems, "lack of money" is likely to be mentioned frequently.

7. Discussions afterwards can invlove criteria for placing items into particular piles.

8. If you do this activity with several groups, it is possible to transform the ratings into a numerical scale:

>   most serious = 3
>
>   intermediate = 2
>
>   least serious = 1

Add up all the scores (ratings) for each of the items in the set of cards and calculate the averages for the group. You can then compare ratings between groups, such as boys versus girls, or urban versus rural youth. This exercise can also be done by individuals, and averages compared between them.

Pile Sorting: (2) Conducting a Grouping Exercise

1. The same cards can be used as for the previous exercise.

2. Ask participants, individually, to sort the cards into groups that are similar, or belong together in some way.

3. After the sorting, you can ask why items were grouped together, but remember to clarify that there are no right or wrong answers.

4. You may wish to conduct the grouping exercise with different types of people, keeping careful records about how the cards were arranged by the different types of people.

APPENDIX I

SUGGESTED REFERENCES ON QUALITATIVE RESEARCH AND RAPID ASSESSMENT METHODS

Qualitative Research References

Bernard H.R. *Research Methods in Cultural Anthropology,* New York, Sage Publications, 1996.

Campbell O., Cleland J., Collumbien M. and Southwick K. *Social Science Methods for Research on Reproductive Health.* Special Programme of Research, Development and Research Training in Human Reproduction. Geneva, World Health Organization, 1999.

Coreil J. Group interview methods in community health research. *Medical Anthropology,* 1995, 16: 193-210.

Cornwall A. and Jewkes R. What is participatory research? *Social Science and Medicine,* 1995, 41(12): 1667-1676.

Dawson S., Manderson L. and Tallo V. *A Manual for the Use of Focus Groups.* Boston, International Foundation for Developing Countries, 1993.

Debus M. *Methodological Review: The Handbook for Excellence in Focus Group Research.* Washington, D.C., Academy for Educational Development (e-mail: admindc@aed.org), n.d.

Denzin N.K. and Lincoln Y.S., eds., *Handbook of Qualitative Research.* Thousand Oaks, Sage Publications, 1994.

Minichiello V., Aroni R., Timewell E. and Alexander L. *In-Depth Interviewing: Researching People.* Melbourne, Lincoln School of Health Sciences, La Trobe University, Longman Cheshire, 1990.

Morgan D.L., ed., *Successful Focus Groups: Advancing the State of the Art.* Newbury Park, Sage Publications, 1993.

Pelto P. Qualitative data-gathering for reproductive health research. *Social Change,* 1996, 26(3-4): 45-72.

QUARC (Website in English): http://www.quarc.de/english.html.

Van Der Walt H. and Mathews C. How do health service managers respond to qualitative research? *Social Science and Medicine,* 1995, 41(12): 1725-1729.

Yoddumnern-Attig B., Attig G. and Boonchalaksi W. *A Field Manual on Selected Qualitative Research Methods.* Salaya, Thailand, Institute for Population and Social Research, Mahidol University, 1989.

Rapid Assessment References

Agyepong I., Aryee B., Dzikunu H. and Manderson L. *The Malaria Manual: Guidelines for the rapid assessment of social, economic and cultural aspects of malaria.* Methods for Social Research in Tropical Diseases No. 2. UNDP/World Bank/WHO Special Programme for Research & Training in Tropical Diseases. Geneva, World Health Organization, 1995.

Bauman F., Brice G., Craig B., Chou S., Gallus C. and Main L. *Planning Health Communities: A Guide to Doing Community Needs Assessment.* Adelaide, Southern Community Health Research Unit, 1991.

Beebe J. Basic concepts and techniques of rapid appraisal. *Human Organization,* 1995, 54(1): 42-51.

Bennett F.J. Qualitative and quantitative methods: in-depth or rapid assessment? *Social Science and Medicine,* 1995, 40(12): 1589-1590.

Gittelsohn J., Anliker J., Davis S., Evans M., Helitzer-Allen D., McCarthy P., Metcalfe L., Sharma A. and Story M. *Formative Assessment Protocol.* Washington, D.C., Pathways Project, 1994.

Gittelsohn J., Pelto P.J., Bentley M.E., Bhattacharya K. and Jensen J.L. *Rapid Assessment Procedures (RAP): Ethnographic Methods to Investigate Women's Health.* Cambridge, MA, International Nutrition Foundation, 1998.

Helitzer-Allen D. and Allen H.A. *The Manual for Targeted Intervention Research on Sexually Transmitted Illnesses with Community Members.* Washington, D.C., Hubert Allen and Associates for Family Health International, 1994.

ILO/UNICEF. *How to Find Out about Child Labour (Quickly).* Geneva, International Labour Organization, 1995.

Larson A. and Manderson L. *Contextual Assessment Procedures for STDs and HIV/AIDS Prevention Programmes: A Manual.* Brisbane, Australian Centre for International and Tropical Health and Nutrition, The University of Queensland, 1995.

Manderson L. and Aaby P. An epidemic in the field? Rapid assessment procedures and health research. *Social Science and Medicine,* 1992a, 35(7): 839-850.

Manderson L. and Aaby P. Can rapid anthropological procedures be applied to tropical diseases? *Health Policy and Planning,* 1992b, 7(1): 46-55.

Nichter M. Introduction. *Medical Anthropology,* 1994, 15: 319-334.

Scrimshaw N.S. and Gleason G.R., eds., *Rapid Assessment Procedures.* Boston, International Nutrition Foundation for Developing Countries, 1992.

Scrimshaw S. and Hurtado E. *Rapid Assessment Procedures for Nutrition and Primary Health Care: Anthropological Approaches to Improving Programme Effectiveness.* Los Angeles, UCLA Latin American Center Publications, University of California, 1987.

United Nations Population Fund (UNFPA). *Population and Reproductive Health Programmes: Applying Rapid Anthropological Assessment Procedures.* Technical Report No. 39. New York, United Nations Population Fund, 1997.

World Health Organization. *Rapid Evaluation Method Guidelines for Maternal and Child Health, Family Planning and Other Health Services.* Division of Family Health & Division of Epidemiological Surveillance and Health Situation and Trend Assessment. Geneva, WHO, 1993.

APPENDIX II

WORKSHOP PROGRAMME TO DEVELOP A RAPID ASSESSMENT PROTOCOL

Introduction

In Part I we discussed in detail the necessary steps to develop a rapid assessment protocol and prepare for fieldwork. We offer here a generic example of a 10-day workshop schedule for undertaking these tasks. The process will be faster for experienced researchers and slower for others, so this should be used flexibly. You may wish to spend relatively more or less time on each component described here, or delete some, or add others. The workshop should be led by a facilitator (e.g. Team leader or an experienced researcher).

The schedule here was used, with moderately experienced teams, in Viet Nam and China. You will see reference to practical sessions. In each location, a Community Meeting was held, both for genuine data gathering and as an opportunity to practise this tool for the field. Youths were also invited to practise free listing and social mapping. All references to Boxes and Steps refer to Part I of the manual.

The crucial objectives of the workshop are:

- Establishing rapport and sense of team cohesion
- Gaining familiarity with the manual and methods (additional practice with unfamiliar tools)
- Making essential basic decisions about sampling, location, methods, time-frame, areas of responsibility, and logistic preparation for fieldwork

Day 1

Morning
- Self-introduction, including interests and past research experience
- Overview of Rapid Assessments and reasons for this assessment
- Brief introduction to the manual

Afternoon
- Discussion of workshop objectives
- Explaining tasks
    - check-lists and question guides for each method
    - preliminary decisions about sampling and location
- Drafting invitation letter to Community Meeting, identifying participants; send letter

Day 2

Morning
- Preparation for fieldwork discussion
    - Community Meetings: purpose
    - Understanding stakeholders and gatekeepers
    - Importance of participatory methods
    - Training of youth/research assistants

Afternoon
- Discussion about 'adolescence' using Box 2 (discussion tool) to generate theme list (Step 3)
- Discussion of sampling issues – the need for diversity
- Invite youth for Day 4 (use local contacts to find them) and prepare small gifts

Day 3

Morning
- Free lists and ratings: how to use them (practical session within the Research Team)
- Social mapping as a tool for FGDs (practical session within Team, e.g. map activities in Ministry of Health central building)

Afternoon
- Mapping for researcher familiarization: how is it used?
- Observation: how, where and what is appropriate to the assessment?
- Collaboration for fieldwork: opportunities and potential problems
- Discuss and plan youth activity for tomorrow
    How will the group be divided?
    What questions will be used for free listing?
    Determining responsibility for organizing materials, rooms, timekeeping, free-listing, ratings, social mapping and discussion, welcoming, thanking

Day 4

Morning
- Youth arrive to do:
    Free listing and rating
    Social mapping and group discussion

Afternoon
- Discuss morning activity
- Discuss/practise data management using morning's data

Day 5

Morning
- Review other methods as necessary (may take some time depending on expertise of Research Team)
- Analysis (overview of basic principles)
- Review of secondary data (types, sources, limitations, use at outset of Assessment and as background for final report)
- Interpretation and synthesis from several data sources (concept of 'triangulation')

Afternoon
- Limitations of rapid assessments
- Prepare for Community Meeting
    - Deciding venue for small group discussions (if any), responsibility for welcoming, explaining exercise, facilitating, synthesizing, thanking
    - Responsibility for materials and refreshments
    - Decisions on discussion topics for small groups, if appropriate

Day 6

Morning
- Community Meeting

Afternoon
- Discuss morning activity
    - Limitations
    - Lessons learnt
    - Thinking about Community Meetings at district or village level
    - Data management
    - Findings: issues, key informants identified

Day 7

Morning
- Ethical and confidentiality issues
- Reassessment of theme list following Community Meeting

Afternoon
- Brainstorming methods to explore themes and issues (see Step 4)
- Work in small groups to develop Check-lists and Question Guides for each method (see Step 5)

Day 8

Morning
- Continue unfinished work from previous afternoon, if any
- Divide into small groups to work on site plans for each area
    Deciding about sampling, methods and approaches to field communication and monitoring, areas of responsibility, time-frame (see Steps 6, 7 & 8)

Afternoon
- Continue work from morning

Day 9

Morning
- Discuss preparation of final report following assessment (see Step 9)

Afternoon
- Time for clarification, reflection, planning

Day 10

Morning
- Finalize theme list, proposed methodology, check-lists and guides (Steps 3-5)
- Finalize time lines and activities (Step 6 & 7)

Afternoon
- Clarification of any issues at request of Team members
- Feedback and evaluation of workshop